AN INTRODUCTION TO RISK PREDICTION
AND PREVENTIVE DENTISTRY

THE AXELSSON SERIES
ON PREVENTIVE DENTISTRY

The world-renowned authority on preventive and community dentistry presents his life's work in this five-volume series of clinical atlases focusing on risk prediction of dental caries and periodontal disease and on needs-related preventive and maintenance programs.

Volume 1   An Introduction to Risk Prediction and Preventive Dentistry
Provides a general overview of current and future trends in risk prediction, control, and nonaggressive management of caries and periodontal disease; preventive dentistry methods and programs; and quality control.

Volume 2   Diagnosis and Risk Prediction of Dental Caries
Includes a comprehensive discussion of the etiology, pathogenesis, diagnosis, risk indicators and factors, individual risk profiles, and epidemiology of caries.

Volume 3   Diagnosis and Risk Prediction of Periodontal Diseases
Presents a comprehensive discussion of the etiology, pathogenesis, diagnosis, risk indicators and factors, individual risk profiles, and epidemiology of periodontal diseases. Considers periodontal diseases as a possible risk factor for systemic diseases and presents current and future trends in the management of periodontal diseases, including nonaggressive debridement and preservation of the root cementum.

Volume 4   Preventive Materials, Methods, and Programs
Discusses self-care and professional methods of mechanical and chemical plaque control, use of fluorides and fissure sealants, and integrated caries prevention. Addresses needs-related preventive programs based on risk prediction and computer-aided epidemiology analysis for quality control and outcome.

Volume 5   Nonaggressive Treatment, Arrest, and Control of Periodontal Diseases and Dental Caries
Details current and future trends in nonaggressive treatment methods that seek to preserve the root cementum; surgical versus nonsurgical periodontal therapy; repair and regeneration of periodontal support; management of furcation-involved teeth; restricted use of antibiotics; arrest of noncavitated enamel, dentin, and root carious lesions; nonaggressive mini-preparations; esthetic and hygienic aspects of restorations; and management of erosions. Focuses on needs-related maintenance programs to ensure the long-term success of treatment and to prevent recurrence of periodontal disease and dental caries.

AN INTRODUCTION TO RISK PREDICTION
AND PREVENTIVE DENTISTRY

Per Axelsson, DDS, Odont Dr

Professor and Chairman
Department of Preventive Dentistry
Public Dental Health Service

Karlstad, Sweden

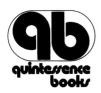

Quintessence Publishing Co, Inc
Chicago, Berlin, London, Tokyo, Paris, Barcelona, São Paulo,
Moscow, Prague, and Warsaw

To my wife Ingrid, my daughter Eva, and my son Torbjörn

Library of Congress Cataloging-in-Publication Data

Axelsson, Per, D.D.S., Odont. Dr.
      An introduction to risk prediction and preventive dentistry / Per
Axelsson.
                        p.   cm. – (The Axelsson series on preventive dentistry ; vol.
1)
      Includes bibliographical references and index.
      ISBN 0-86715-361-X
      1. Preventive dentistry.   2. Dental caries—Prevention.
3. Periodontal disease—Prevention. I. Title. II. Title: Risk
prediction and preventive dentistry. III. Series: Axelsson, Per,
D.D.S. Axelsson series on preventive dentistry ; vol. 1.
      [DNLM: 1. Dental Caries—prevention & control. 2. Periodontal
Diseases—prevention & control. 3. Preventive Dentistry. 4. Risk
Factors. WU 270 A969i 2000]
RK60.7.A94 2000
617.6—dc21
DNLM/DLC
for Library of Congress   99-16511
                                                                    CIP

© 1999 Quintessence Publishing Co, Inc

Quintessence Publishing Co, Inc
551 Kimberly Drive
Carol Stream, Illinois 60188

Editor: Cheryl Anderson-Wiedenbeck
Production: Gerda Steinmeyer

Printed in Germany

CONTENTS

Contents

PREFACE

The etiology of dental caries and periodontal diseases is well understood, and we have now developed efficient methods for preventing these diseases. Over the last 25 years in County of Värmland, Sweden, large-scale implementation of our prevention programs has led to an increase in the percentage of caries-free 3 year olds, from 30% to 97%, while reducing caries in 12 year olds from an average of 25 DFS to less than 1 (0.6). In the last 10 years, we have increased the number of remaining teeth in 65 year olds by more than 15% and reduced their loss of periodontal support by more than 20%, at the same time reducing the percentage who are edentulous from 17% to 7%.

According to the principles of *lege artis*, all members of our profession are obliged to offer treatment based on the most current scientific and clinical knowledge available. As we enter the new millennium, we must therefore continue to concentrate our efforts on preventing, controlling, and arresting the development of dental caries and periodontal diseases. However, needs-related preventive and maintenance programs must be cost effective and should be based on information derived from comprehensive diagnoses, histories, and risk predictions at group, individual, and tooth surface levels. For quality control and evaluation of such programs, computer-aided analytical epidemiology, using relevant variables, should be introduced.

The aim of this clinical textbook and atlas is to provide a broad overview of current and future trends in oral health care resources, diagnosis, risk prediction, prevention, and "nonaggressive" treatment of dental caries and periodontal diseases. This book, the first volume of a five-volume series, should also serve as an "appetizer" to the more comprehensive clinical textbooks and atlases to come, in which a detailed scientific background, a well illustrated guide to implementing the "state of the art," and conclusions and future recommendations will be provided for each topic addressed. Thus the series will be useful not only for dentists and dental hygienists, but also for undergraduate and postgraduate students and teachers.

This project could not have been completed without the assistance and support of my family, friends, and colleagues. I offer my deepest thanks to my wife Ingrid and my daughter Eva and son Torbjörn and their families, as well as to all my other relatives and friends, for their patience and understanding throughout the last 5 years in which I spent almost every night, weekend, and vacation preparing the material for these five volumes. I also wish to thank my wonderful staff at the Department of Preventive Dentistry, Public Dental Health Service, County of Värmland, for all their service, and particularly my assistant, Pia Hird, who typed most of my manuscript. I owe special thanks to Art Director Fredrik Persson, Dr Jörgen Paulander, and the Dumex Company for their excellent support with computer-aided illustrations, and to Associate Professor Joan Bevenius for her work in checking my English manuscript.

I am very grateful to all my colleagues and friends around the world and to several publishers (Munksgaard International, The American Academy of Periodontology, S. Karger Medical and Scientific Publisher, FDI World Dental Press, WHO Oral Health Unit), who have generously permitted me to use their illustrations (about 20% of the total). Last but not least, the excellent cooperation of the publisher is gratefully acknowledged.

CHAPTER 1

WORLDWIDE PREVALENCE OF ORAL DISEASE

ORAL HEALTH TRENDS

In many industrialized and several developing countries, 30% to 50% of the population older than 65 years is edentulous (40% in the United States; almost 60% in the United Kingdom). In many 50 to 65 year olds , most of the molars—the most efficient teeth for chewing—have been lost. Among 35 to 50 year olds in many industrialized countries, 35 to 50 tooth surfaces are restored with esthetically unacceptable materials, such as amalgam or gold. However, among adults in many industrialized countries, the percentage of edentulous people has decreased and the number of remaining teeth has increased in recent decades. Several factors have shaped oral health trends globally, affecting the rates of caries and periodontal disease.

Caries prevalence

Caries prevalence has decreased significantly among children and young adults in most industrialized countries during the last two decades. Every year since 1969, the World Health Organization (WHO) has compiled a world map of caries prevalence at age 12 years, expressed as the number of decayed, missing, or filled teeth (DMFT) (WHO's Oral Health Unit Data Bank, 1994) Among 12 year olds , the 5-level scale varies from 0.0 to 6.6 DMFT (Table 1).

Figures 1 and 2 show the global maps of caries prevalence in 12 year olds in 1969 and in 1993, respectively. In 1969, the overall picture showed sharp contrasts: The mean number of DMFT was very high, high, or moderate (from 2.7 to > 6.5) in industrialized countries, and generally very low, low, and occasionally moderate in developing countries.

Table 1 Five-level scale of caries prevalence, expressed as the number of decayed, missing, or filled teeth (DMFT)

Color on map*	Level	DMFT
Green	Very low caries prevalence	0.0–1.1
Blue	Low caries prevalence	1.2–2.6
Yellow	Moderate prevalence	2.7–4.4
Red	High prevalence	4.5–6.5
Brown	Very high caries prevalence	> 6.5

* See Figs 1 and 2.

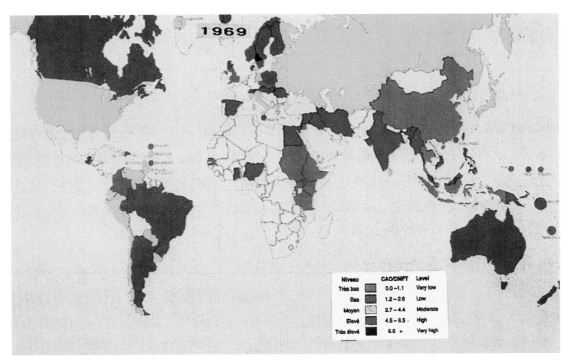

Fig 1 Worldwide caries prevalence among 12 year olds in 1969. (From WHO, 1994. Reprinted with permission.)

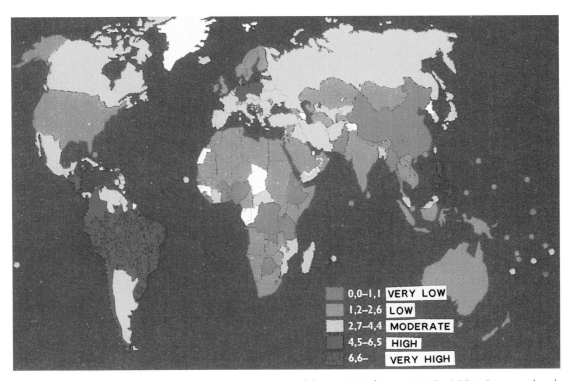

Fig 2 Worldwide caries prevalence among 12 year olds in 1993. (From WHO, 1994. Reprinted with permission.)

Fig 3 Change in caries prevalence among 12 year olds living in the county of Värmland, Sweden, 1964 to 1994. (DFS) Decayed or filled surface.

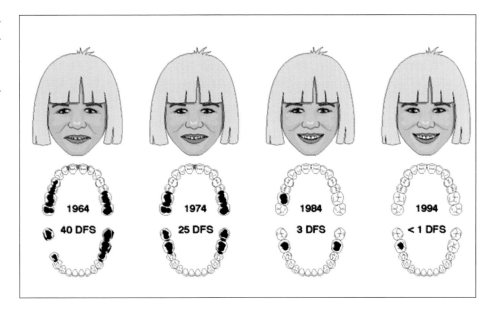

Over the next two decades, there was a downward movement and sometimes a spectacular drop in the prevalence of caries in virtually all the industrialized countries. In particular, the Scandinavian countries, Australia, and New Zealand improved from very high to low caries prevalence. Regionally, some areas improved even more dramatically, as did the county of Värmland in southwestern Sweden, from one of the highest prevalences of caries in the world to a very low prevalence (< 1 decayed or filled surface [DFS]) (Fig 3). In developing countries, the general trend is for caries prevalence to increase, except where preventive programs have been set up.

What lies behind the spectacular drop in caries prevalence in some countries? How can the prevalence be prevented from rising again? How can the deteriorating situation in other countries be halted? The answer to all three questions is one and the same: *prevention, more prevention, and still more prevention.*

In industrialized countries, the promotion of oral hygiene, the widespread use of fluoride toothpastes, the introduction of fluoride into drinking water or salt in some countries, and the availability of advice on nutrition (no sweets between meals, etc) are the factors behind an unprecedented public health success story.

Apart from the fluoridation of water, salt, and milk, which requires more advanced technology and supervised central administration, the aforementioned methods use simple techniques, cost little, and are perfectly suited to implementation at the primary level of health care. As a result of the progress made in the last 25 years, developing countries now have the knowledge and means of prevention to enable them to avoid the costly problems that industrialized countries have had to face and indeed are still facing.

Dental care, as we practice it, is categorized as follows:

1. "Primary" primary prevention. Preventive dentistry measures provided to all pregnant women to prevent postnatal transmission of cariogenic microbes and poor dietary habits from mother to child, etc.
2. Primary prevention. Maintenance of the intact dentition, ie, prevention of dental caries, gingivitis, and periodontitis in a "100%" healthy mouth.

Table 2 Distributions of dental care provided to children and young adults (aged 0 to 19 years) in the county of Värmland, Sweden

Decade	"Primary" primary prevention	Primary prevention	Secondary prevention	Tertiary prevention	Relief of pain
1900–1930	0%	0%	0%	25%	75%
1930–1950	0%	0%	2%	48%	50%
1950–1960	0%	0%	10%	70%	20%
1960–1970	0%	5%	20%	70%	5%
1970–1980	5%	15%	40%	40%	0%
1980–1990	15%	45%	30%	10%	0%

3. Secondary prevention. Prevention from recurrence of disease (dental caries, gingivitis, and periodontitis) after successful symptomatic treatment.
4. Tertiary prevention. Symptomatic treatment of dental caries, gingivitis, and periodontitis, ie, restorations, scaling, and periodontal surgery.
5. Relief of pain. Extractions and endodontic treatment.

Table 2 shows the distribution of the different forms of dental care for children and young adults in the county of Värmland, Sweden, from 1900 to 1990; the increasing rates of early preventive efforts explain the dramatic reduction in the number of DFSs in 12 year olds from 1964 to 1994 (see Fig 3) (Axelsson et al, 1993).

Periodontal disease prevalence

There are few international surveys on the prevalence of periodontal diseases expressed in loss of periodontal support (probing attachment loss). The Community Periodontal Index of Treatment Needs (CPITN) was recommended in the early 1980s by a joint working group from the WHO and the Fédération Dentaire Internationale (Ainamo et al, 1982). The CPITN records four clinical signs of periodontal diseases (Fig 4):

1. Bleeding gingiva
2. Calculus
3. Shallow periodontal pockets (4 to 5 mm)
4. Deep periodontal pockets (> 5 mm)

A periodontal pocket is considered to be present when the gingiva, under the effect of inflammation and/or infection, retracts, forms a pocket, and no longer adheres to the tooth. The ligaments become impaired and the tooth becomes increasingly loose.

To measure periodontal status, the mouth is divided into six parts, or sextants. A specially designed probe is used to test the condition of the gingiva around the tooth selected as the index tooth for each sextant. If several clinical signs are present simultaneously, the most severe is selected.

The WHO has compiled data on more than 100 surveys carried out in individuals aged 35 to 44 years (Miyazaki et al, 1991a, 1991b, 1992). These data should be treated with caution, because very few of the surveys provide a national estimate. In addition, our own data show that treatment needs indicated by the CPITN are greatly overestimated

Fig 4 Clinical signs of peri-odontal disease recorded by the Community Periodontal Index of Treatment Needs.

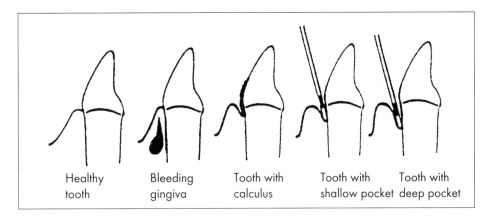

Healthy tooth

Bleeding gingiva

Tooth with calculus

Tooth with shallow pocket

Tooth with deep pocket

at the sextant, and even the tooth, level compared to the surface level, that is, the "true" treatment need. Nevertheless, the data are of great interest because they consistently show a similar pattern of frequency and severity of involvement, which challenges some generally accepted ideas about the distribution and the etiologic process of periodontal disease.

The data show that the percentage of people who have deep pockets (> 5 mm) and the mean number of sextants per person displaying deep pockets are low to very low; ie, the severe forms of periodontal disease, requiring complicated treatment, are far from common (Miyazaki et al, 1991a, 1991b, 1992). Moreover, there seems to be no difference in frequency between industrialized countries and developing countries for the severe forms of periodontal disease. On the other hand, the initial forms (bleeding and calculus) are much more prevalent in developing countries because fewer dental care resources are available and oral hygiene habits are poorer.

In light of these data, it may be stated that generalized periodontal destruction is rare in 40-year-old adults (Miyazaki et al, 1991b). Where some signs of such destruction are present, only a limited part of the dentition is affected. Except in a minority of patients, the initial forms (bleeding and calculus) do not seem to progress inevitably

to the advanced stages of the disease (Norderyd et al, 1999).

ORAL DISEASE PREVENTION

Changing attitudes toward teeth

If the goal of oral health care is to maintain a natural dentition throughout life, the loss of all teeth is the ultimate failure, closely followed by the high percentage of people with only 20 or fewer remaining teeth. The relevant question is why such a high failure rate has been accepted by the public and the dental profession. Intact teeth and healthy gingiva are simply beautiful, attractive, functional parts of the body and should be much more highly regarded by the population. On the other hand, carious teeth, swollen, red, bleeding gingiva, and bad breath are most unattractive.

Under similar conditions, patients would never accept destruction of other parts of the body: An ugly false nose, breasts, or other parts of the body normally covered by clothes would never be accepted. Why should they accept false teeth? Patients would not accept having even 1%

of the nose replaced by amalgam or gold. Imagine having to amputate a finger once every 5 years and replace it with a gold finger, in spite of regular checkups once or twice a year, because of an infectious disease—in an age when this disease, with a well-known etiology, could be successfully prevented.

It is the duty of dental professionals to educate and motivate the public, health personnel, and politicians to regard intact teeth and healthy gingiva as highly as, for example, a healthy nose, eyes, or ears and a justifiable external mode of dress. It is all a matter of changing attitudes and priorities. Famous clothing designers change fashions annually, and people accept the extra costs without hesitation.

A healthy and well-cared for mouth facilitates communication and human relationships. In addition, the boost in health, well being, and self-confidence not only is very important for quality of life but also contributes at a very basic biologic level to protection from systemic infection and other damage. For example, recent analytical studies have disclosed a clear relationship between periodontal diseases and cardiovascular diseases (see Beck et al, 1996, for a review). Therefore, when oral health is compromised, overall health and quality of life are also compromised.

Patient responsibility

Motivation is defined as readiness to act or the driving force behind our actions. Greater responsibility has been described as the motivating factor of longest duration. Optimized responsibility may sometimes result in lifelong motivation, in contrast to the limited durations of encouragement provided by, for example, commendation or a salary increase.

Adults should believe, "No dentist or dental hygienist should accept more responsibility for my oral status than I do myself, because it is my mouth." However, in many industrialized countries with well-organized social health and wel-

fare systems, the population is more or less passive; patients regard the dentist and dental hygienist as responsible for their oral health, the physician as responsible for their general health, and the politicians as responsible for their social welfare.

With the current level of knowledge about the etiology, prevention, and control of dental caries and periodontal diseases, it has been shown that patients who are well motivated and well educated in self-diagnosis and self-care can prevent and control these diseases by themselves. Much more important to general health, quality of life, and costs for health and welfare are the following examples: It is estimated that, among external (environmental) carcinogenic factors, an unhealthy diet accounts for about 30% of cancers, smoking for about 20%, and viruses for about 10%. (The simple message on diet is reduction of animal fat and increased intake of fiber-rich vegetables and fruits, which are the cheapest and most accessible food products in tropical and subtropical climates, where most of the world population lives.) For cardiovascular diseases, unhealthy diet and smoking, along with physical inactivity, are also highly ranked as external (environmental) risk factors. Physical inactivity may also result in skeletal disasters, particularly back pain. The important question is: "Who is responsible for what you eat, whether you smoke, or whether you exercise?" Health maintained and controlled by self-diagnosis and self-care is not only cost effective, but also an important factor in quality of life to maintain independence and health.

Practitioner responsibility

The *lege artis* principles require clinicians to practice dentistry according to modern science and established, well-tried methods, ie, the state of the art. From experimental and well-controlled longitudinal clinical studies in humans, the following conclusions may be drawn about etiologic and modifying factors of dental caries and periodontal diseases and efficient preventive methods (see Axelsson, 1994, 1998, for reviews):

1. Dental caries and periodontal diseases can successfully be prevented and controlled by self-care supplemented by needs-related professional preventive measures.
2. Carious lesions affecting enamel, root, and even dentin can be arrested successfully.
3. Regeneration of periodontal attachment is a reality.

According to the *lege artis* principles, the profession is obliged to concentrate on prevention, control, and arrest of dental caries and periodontal diseases. For dental caries, "prevention instead of extension" or at least "prevention before extension," should be given priority. By the same token, aggressive treatment of dental caries with extractions and "drilling, filling, and billing," and of periodontal diseases with extractions, aggressive scaling, and extensive flap surgery, must be regarded as outdated and more or less unjustified.

CONCLUSION

Oral health and general health are strongly correlated with the level of education. All over the world, the level of education is improving. Eventually, increasingly well-educated patients will learn the implications of high-quality dentistry according to *lege artis* principles and will request more preventive dentistry, instead of "drilling, filling, and billing." Dentists who are not willing to comply with their patients' requests will find that their practices decline.

CHAPTER 2

GLOBAL ORAL HEALTH CARE RESOURCES

ORAL HEALTH PERSONNEL

Ratio of oral health personnel to population

During the last two decades, there has been a dramatic decrease in the previously high levels of dental caries among children in most industrialized countries (WHO's Oral Health Unit Data Bank, 1994). In many developing countries, however, caries prevalence has increased from previous low levels. In addition, the prevalence of mod-

erate periodontal treatment needs (Community Periodontal Index of Treatment Needs [CPITN] scores 1 to 3) is much higher in developing countries than in industrialized countries, despite a similar prevalence of advanced periodontal treatment needs (CPITN score 4). However, the dilemma is that the developing countries represent the absolute majority of the world's population.

Figure 5 shows the percentage of the world's population by World Health Organization (WHO) regions in 1986. Asia alone (SEARO and WPRO) contains more than 50% of the world's

Fig 5 World population by World Health Organization regions. (EURO) Regional Office for Europe; (EMRO) Regional Office for the Eastern Mediterranean; (AMRO) Regional Office for the Americas; (AFRO) Regional Office for Africa; (WPRO) Regional Office for the Western Pacific; (SEARO) Regional Office for Southeast Asia. (Modified from WHO, 1986.)

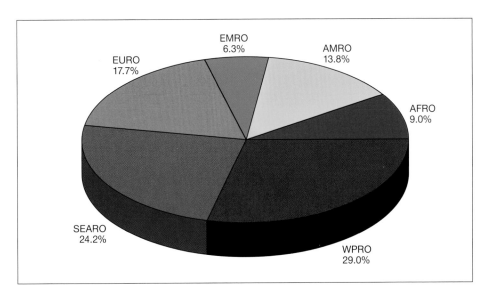

9

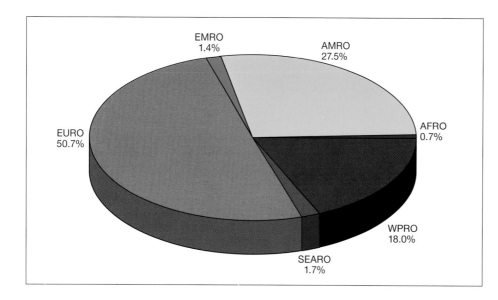

Fig 6 Oral health personnel by World Health Organization regions. (EURO) Regional Office for Europe; (EMRO) Regional Office for the Eastern Mediterranean; (AMRO) Regional Office for the Americas; (AFRO) Regional Office for Africa; (WPRO) Regional Office for the Western Pacific; (SEARO) Regional Office for Southeast Asia. (Modified from WHO, 1986.)

population. China and India alone have more than 2.3 billion inhabitants (40%). According to WHO's Data Bank in 1986, Europe has more than 50% of the world's oral health personnel resources (dentists, dental hygienists, dental assistants, technicians, etc) (Fig 6), although it has only 17.7% of the world's population (see Fig 5). The extremes of the ratio of dentists to inhabitants are found in Scandinavia (1:1,000) and in China and India (1:120,000).

Increasing the availability of oral health personnel

Improving dental schools worldwide

Overcoming this imbalance in the ratio of oral health personnel, particularly of dentists, to the population in different countries is a major challenge. Many developing countries are experiencing either an actual increase in caries prevalence or an inability to reduce the existing level. Although the disease prevalence is, or threatens to be, only moderate, its impact is much more seri-

ous than would be the case in industrialized countries, because of the almost total lack of effective care.

These countries have responded to the problem by attempting to develop new dental schools with curricula adapted from those that were common, but are now changing, in industrialized countries. More serious still is the fact that, irrespective of which curricula these countries may have chosen, there is a crippling lack of qualified teaching staff. In practical terms, this shortfall results in failure to deliver, often by a wide margin, whatever curricula are offered in faculty handbooks.

This predicament is not limited to developing countries. There is a wide divergence of dental school performance across the range of industrialized countries and within any country in which there are a number of dental schools. Even where schools may be judged to be similar in quality, strength and creativity may vary markedly from subject to subject. The profession is thus facing a challenge to minimize undesirable variation and to provide up-to-date and high-quality education for all.

An answer lies in broad exploitation of new communication skills, which are so versatile in keeping information at hand and in offering opportunities for interactive use by undergraduates and graduates as well as teaching staff. An obvious outcome will be the development of a new type of student as well as new types of teachers. Major elements of this new experience will be:

1. Much greater ease in pooling intellectual resources
2. Speedy exchange of information, especially in relation to effective new methodologies and materials
3. Development of common assessment methods
4. Access to a wide variety of databanks
5. Greater opportunity to remodel careers over extended periods of time according to the speed of change in society and the job market

Preparation of a broad set of modules, serving the oral health stream within a health sciences structure, will demonstrate what might be achieved and thus initiate a snowballing effect toward the ultimate objective of a complete computer-assisted curriculum. Already there are several centers of excellence around the globe producing the type of interactive materials needed for computer-assisted training. The assortment of such programs is steadily increasing and available as CD-ROM and on the Internet. There is a need to direct that excellence toward the overall objective. This is what the WHO hopes to do, in collaboration with the International Federation of Dental Education Associations, which is enthusiastic about this approach (WHO Oral Health Unit, 1994).

Succinctly, empowerment of the learner is the principal aim of this concept, in both a variation on the theme of universities without walls and an attempt to make excellence available whatever the constraints of quantity and quality in teaching staff. It will benefit dental schools where resources needed to deliver an adequate and appropriate curriculum are very scarce. Every school will need a certain core of staff to administer, coordinate, guide, evaluate, and conduct practical exercises. The specific teaching and

learning, however, would come largely from the student, the graduate, and the teachers interacting with the computer programs at their disposal. The excellence of those programs would depend on having a "braintrust" group of the very best experts responsible for devising the programs. In this way the best available courses would be offered to all students, everywhere, rather than the wide range of messages, often contradictory or outdated, that students currently receive.

Whatever the definitive choice of approaches, an initiative of this type will streamline the training of health personnel, with sufficient flexibility to ensure that training of health personnel will keep pace with the leading edge of science more clearly than is the case today.

Expanding the role of dental hygienists

However, in many countries, the need for dental treatment is overwhelming for the low ratio of dentists, particularly in developing countries in Asia, Africa, and Latin America, which are home to the majority of the world's population. There is a clear indication for training of dental hygienists, who are committed exclusively to prevention and control of dental caries and periodontal diseases and periodontal treatment. In addition, their work is very cost effective (Axelsson et al, 1991, Axelsson, 1998).

The role and supply of dental hygienists are of increasing interest worldwide, mainly because of a growing acknowledgment of the importance of oral health as a part of general health, renewed emphasis on setting and attaining health policy goals, and recognition of dental hygienists as a major resource for attaining those goals. Dental hygienists today constitute one of the largest and fastest growing groups in oral health service. They practice, in collaboration with other health professionals, primarily as clinicians and health educators. Their work involves the use of preventive and therapeutic methods to promote good health and to prevent and control oral diseases.

According to Fédération Dentaire Internationale surveys (FDI, 1990), dental hygienists are

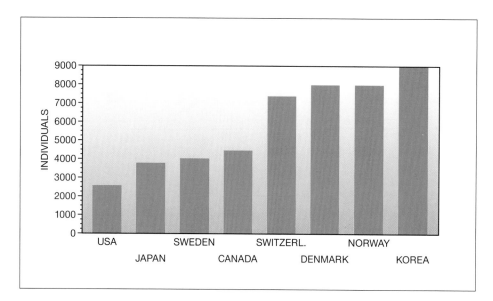

Fig 7 Population per dental hygienist.

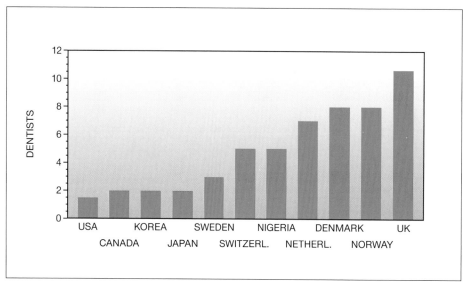

Fig 8 Dentists per dental hygienist.

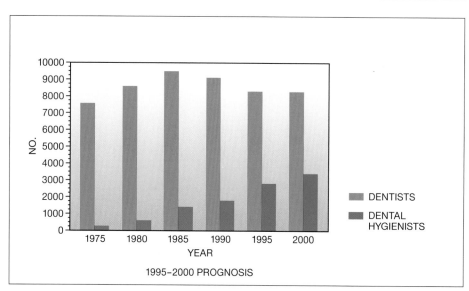

Fig 9 Dentists and dental hygienists in Sweden.

now trained in more than 25 countries. The pioneers were the United States (1906), followed by Norway (1924), Great Britain (1943), Canada (1947), Japan (1949), Nigeria (1958), and Sweden and the Netherlands (1968). The United States has the highest ratio of dental hygienists per head of population (1:2,500), followed by Japan, Sweden, and Canada (about 1:4,000) (Fig 7). The United States also has the highest ratio of dental hygienists to dentists (0.75:1), followed by Japan (0.5:1), South Korea (0.5:1), Canada (0.5:1), and Sweden (0.3:1) (Fig 8). Figure 9 shows the ratio of dental hygienists to dentists in Sweden retrospectively from 1975 and prospectively to 2000 (Axelsson et al, 1993b).

In most countries, the length of the dental hygienist-training program is 2 years, but it may range from 1 to 4 years. The entrance requirement is qualification as a dental assistant or matriculation from high school. The occupation is held predominantly by women (more than 90%).

According to a survey in 13 countries (Australia, Canada, Denmark, Italy, Japan, Korea, the Netherlands, Nigeria, Norway, Sweden, Switzerland, Great Britain, and the United States), which covers most of the world's dental hygienists, the legal scope of their clinical practice is remarkably similar (FDI, 1990). It is characterized by a common set of procedures and activities, including treatment planning for the dental hygiene stages of care; history taking on general health, socioeconomic, and oral health aspects; provision of optimized self-care for individuals and groups; scaling; root planing; debridement and professional mechanical tooth cleaning; topical application of fluoride gels and varnishes; use of fissure sealants; finishing of restorations and removal of overhangs; dietary evaluations and counseling; and administration of salivary and oral microbiology tests. In some countries, including Sweden, the training program also emphasizes behavioral science. Dental hygienists are also trained in local anesthesia (infiltration and regional block).

In Sweden, the training program for dental assistants also includes practical preventive dentistry. They are responsible for most of the preventive measures so successfully carried out in children and young adults. Because the training program takes less than half the time required for the dental hygiene program, this personnel category could well be appropriate in other countries.

Oral health personnel in retrospect

For too long, the oral cavity has been separated from the rest of body and "donated" to dentists, a profession more or less independent from the general medical professions. At the beginning of this century, dentistry centered around extraction of teeth and making complete and partial dentures, with the assistance of technicians. Then came an era of "drilling, filling, and billing" in most industrialized countries and "aggressive" exploration of the tooth crown because of dental caries. In recent decades, in many industrialized countries, the roots of the teeth have also been exploited by subspecialists in periodontology and endodontics, and teeth have been moved around for functional and esthetic reasons by specialists in orthodontics.

Recently, successful reconstruction with implant technology has been achieved through the teamwork of oral surgeons, periodontists, prosthodontists, and dental technicians. Specialists in periodontology now offer regeneration of periodontal support.

Oral health personnel of the future

Integrated education

According to the *lege artis* principles, modern knowledge and experience obliges dental professionals to focus on prevention and control of dental caries, periodontal diseases, and other oral diseases concurrently with elimination of existing treatment needs.

Increasing numbers of individuals worldwide will have intact tooth crowns and no loss of periodontal support. Therefore, the tooth crowns and the roots have to be reunited in the oral cavity, and the oral cavity must be returned to its rightful place in the body. This requires a more holistic approach, centered on the owner of the oral cavity. Preventive dentistry and oral health promotion have to be integrated with general health promotion, in collaboration with general health personnel. Dental education has to be comprehensively reoriented to serve the changing needs of oral health, linked more closely to the requirements of the whole health sector.

As an alternative to existing schools, which are specific to medicine, dentistry, nursing, and pharmacy, the aim should be to create an integrated system for educating all health personnel within a health sciences school structure. Elimination of separate training of auxiliary and professional personnel categories is also desirable. A "ladder" system of education is envisaged, in which, for the oral health stream, the "oral physician," instead of today's dentist, is seen as the highest level category, at parity with the other medical specialties. Other oral health personnel categories, such as dental assistants, prophylaxis dental assistants, and dental hygienists would leave this ladder at various levels, corresponding to defined lists of duties, as would be the case for personnel focusing on any other health area. A number of dental schools, predominantly but not exclusively in Europe, have already begun to move toward this type of structure.

Integrated health teams

At the community and city levels, integrated local health teams should be established to improve oral health as well as general health among the population. Such a team should consist of well-trained professionals, highly experienced in prevention and health promotion rather than treatment:

1. General physician
2. Psychologist
3. Nutritionist
4. Sociologist
5. Physiotherapist
6. Physical education teacher
7. Engineer
8. Oral physician
9. General health nurse
10. Dental hygienist

The general physician should be the leader of the team. Therefore he or she should be the most highly qualified and experienced in leadership and communication, general medicine, general health promotion, and epidemiology.

The psychologist should be highly qualified and experienced in behavioral science, with special reference to establishing good, healthy lifestyle habits and eliminating bad habits, such as smoking.

The nutritionist should be highly qualified and experienced in the concept of "input and output" related to eating at the cellular level as well as the individual level. Emphasis should be placed on the consequences of healthy versus unhealthy dietary habits.

The sociologist should be well educated and experienced in the influence of socioeconomic conditions on health status.

The physiotherapist should be well educated and experienced in how to prevent the development (primary prevention) and the recurrence (secondary prevention) of musculoskeletal orthopedic problems (back pain, etc) as well as diagnosis and early rehabilitation of such problems.

The physical education teacher should be well educated and experienced in the consequences of physical training and activity versus physical inactivity for general health and how to activate all members of the population.

The engineer should be well educated and experienced in the effects of the external and internal environment on health and how to diagnose and eliminate unhealthy environments.

The oral physician will be the leader of the oral health personnel team and highly qualified and experienced in preventive dentistry and oral health promotion as an integrated part of general health promotion.

The general health nurse will be responsible for education of the population in self-diagnosis and self-care, with special reference to prevention and control of diseases.

The dental hygienist should be well educated and experienced in optimizing oral self-diagnosis and self-care for prevention and control of dental caries, periodontal diseases, and other oral diseases, supplemented by needs-related professional preventive measures.

The local health team should be backed up, at the county level, by a central resource team with a great variety of specialists and subspecialists. Most should have a scientific background at the doctorate (PhD) level:

1. Physicians, all specialties
2. Psychologists
3. Sociologists
4. Nutritionists
5. Oral physicians
6. Epidemiologists
7. Statisticians
8. Economists

The remainder should have extensive research experience:

1. Physiotherapists
2. Sports professionals
3. Engineers
4. General nurses

5. Dental hygienists
6. Public relations officers
   a. Art directors
   b. Copywriters

The effects of such teams on the health status of the population and the costs should be repeatedly evaluated in terms of the following:

1. Absence from work because of disease
2. Internationally (WHO-) accepted, disease-specific variables
3. Cost effectiveness and cost-benefit ratio

ORAL CARE SYSTEMS AND TRENDS

Needs analysis

Public health leaders (ministers of health, chief dental officers, etc) in all countries confront the same challenge: how to design, set up, regularly evaluate and modify services that cover needs and meet demand. To add to the complexity of the task, all decisions are subject to budgetary constraints, which often pay very little attention to genuine public health considerations.

In the oral health field, there is a set of methods enabling each country to analyze the needs, the demand, and the response of the oral health care system. These methods have been developed over the last 20 years, in the course of international collaborative studies (ICSs) on oral health care systems, and promoted by the WHO. The study is performed on a random population sample of each key age group for oral diseases: 12 years, 35 to 44 years, and 65 years and older. The oral health status of each individual is recorded by clinical examination, and the findings are used to calculate the current health status and treatment needs. Moreover, a questionnaire completed by the subjects provides information on attitudes, behavior, level of satisfaction, and other factors relating to demand for and consumption of care.

The study is supplemented by a survey on a sample of the personnel concerned: dentists, dental auxiliaries, dental hygienists, dental assistants, heads of school health services, and so on. In addition to these data on the consumers and providers of care, the study provides structural, macroeconomic, and sociologic data. On completion of an ICS, a full description of the health system of the sector is available, together with an estimate of the levels of disease and the treatment needs. It is thus possible to analyze the weaknesses and strengths of the system and the way in which these are perceived by the population. All these data have to be taken into account whenever it is intended, for example, to introduce a new system of fees, to promote hygiene and prevention programs, or to redesign personnel-training programs.

If repeated periodically, the exercise makes it possible to follow trends in disease, to estimate the growth of demand and treatment coverage, and thus to make the necessary adjustments and plan personnel resources for the coming decades.

Oral diseases differ from one country to another, but only in terms of prevalence or severity, not in kind. The principles of prevention are likewise universal: improved plaque control and controlled use of fluorides through self-care, supplemented by professional care, and a low-sugar diet. Types of treatment comply, theoretically, with the principle that identical problems require an identical response. Despite these similarities, oral health care systems differ markedly from one country to another. It is useful therefore to compare the various systems and to see what aspects, structures, or approaches seem to provide the best response to a given situation.

From 1973 to 1981, ICS-I was conducted in 10 countries representing a wide range of systems from wholly private to wholly public, with a series of intermediate stages—some with school health services, some without—all funded in very different ways. The participating countries were Australia, Canada (Alberta, Ontario, and Quebec), The Federal Republic of Germany, The German Democratic Republic, Ireland, Japan, New Zealand, Norway, Poland, and the United States. Six of these countries took part in ICS-II (1988 to 1993), which permitted a comparison of their situation after about 10 years. They are Germany (Erfurt site), Japan, New Zealand, Poland, and the United States (Baltimore site). They were joined by France and two new sites in the United States. The ICS surveys have made it possible to construct a unique database on oral health systems around the world. This source of information can be a useful aid to planners who wish to evaluate or replan their systems but who lack the necessary resources to carry out an ICS-type study in their own country. The international collaborative studies have had a considerable impact. Some countries have literally discovered their own oral health situation, and some systems have been entirely restructured or redirected as a result. Afterward, ICS-II enabled these countries to measure the progress made. For example, 36% of 40 year olds in New Zealand were completely edentulous at the time of ICS-I, but 15 years later the figure was only 16%.

Experience of the international comparison to date shows that ICSs overturn some generally accepted ideas:

1. Oral health status does not seem to depend on the type of personnel or on access to care.
2. Care provided in the school setting is very effective in the treatment of childhood oral diseases but does not appear to improve the oral health of adults in the long term, except when backed up by the instruction of both patients and oral health personnel in prevention techniques.
3. The most decisive factors for oral health are linked to the ability of oral health personnel and governments to promote prevention activities.

In other words, facilitating access to care and increasing the number of dentists are not necessarily the best responses in the oral health field. When oral health programs are planned, priority should always be given to prevention, whatever the level of resources available, and each situation should be analyzed in its own right and in comparison with others.

Improving access to oral care

Traditional systems for oral care are based on various combinations of public-salaried services and private practice. The public services are usually responsible for prevention and for care of schoolchildren and disadvantaged groups. Private practitioners provide a wide range of treatment to the general public. All these systems are oriented in such a way that the dentist provides most of the care.

The level of dental caries in developing countries has rarely been as high as in industrialized countries, except for Latin America. In some developing countries, successful preventive programs have been implemented. However, in many there is still a threat of increasing caries, related to changing diet and lifestyles in combination with poor oral hygiene and no use of fluoride toothpaste. In many communities, the oral care systems do not meet even the basic needs of the public. Most public services have only very low coverage; communities in low-income rural and urban areas cannot afford private oral care. Further, developing countries cannot afford to establish, staff, and run education facilities for dentists or hope to provide adequate employment opportunities for dentists trained abroad.

In all countries, economic restraints, changes in demand for oral health care, political pressures to extend services to underprivileged groups, and concerns about quality, costs, and effectiveness of care demand that alternative ways of organizing oral health care be examined and implemented. Cost and lack of access for underprivileged and low-income groups constrain all oral health care systems.

What actions can be taken to combat this neglect, break down the barriers of cost, and improve access to oral health care? Alternative oral care systems must be developed so that a maximum number of people can have access to and can afford oral health care. Several recent advances give great scope for the transformation of the delivery and quality of oral care:

1. New educational technologies via interactive training (the Internet, etc) that make learning—both knowledge and skills—simpler and faster for all types of personnel
2. Simplified and logical design of oral clinics that improve the workplace and substantially reduce the capital costs of equipment and the need for maintenance
3. Better materials that are easier and simpler to use

Based on these technological advances, three types of care can be defined:

1. Simple low technology; very cost effective
2. Moderate level of technology; rather expensive
3. High technology; often extremely expensive

The first level of oral care includes education of the population in self-diagnosis and self-care on an individual and a group basis; professional mechanical tooth cleaning; use of fluoride varnish and fissure sealants; scaling, root planing, and debridement; and low-technology treatment of single-surface caries cavities with the so-called atraumatic restorative technique, which has the potential to revolutionize the type of care that can be given in developing countries with a low ratio of dentists.

The atraumatic restorative technique is based on the use of dental hand instruments and glass-ionomer cement, a recently developed dental restorative material. Unlike conventional techniques, the technique does not require electricity or clean piped water to operate equipment. Because glass-ionomer cement adheres very effectively to dental tissues, the carious teeth do not have to be cut and shaped with a dental handpiece, as they do for amalgam restorations. Re-

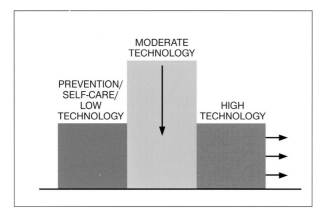

Fig 10 Changes in distribution of tasks in oral health care from past to present in highly industrialized countries. (Modified from WHO, 1994. Reprinted with permission.)

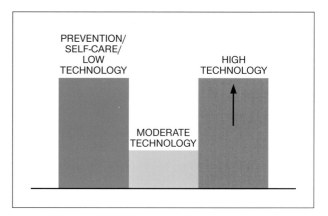

Fig 11 Distribution of tasks in oral health care in highly industrialized countries. (Modified from WHO, 1994. Reprinted with permission.)

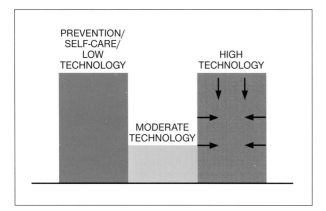

Fig 12 Future distribution of tasks in oral health care in highly industrialized countries. (Modified from WHO, 1994. Reprinted with permission.)

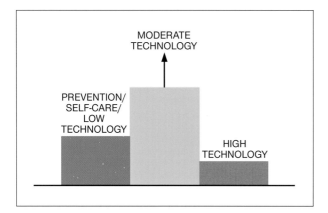

Fig 13 Typical distribution of tasks in oral health care in developing countries. (Modified from WHO, 1994. Reprinted with permission.)

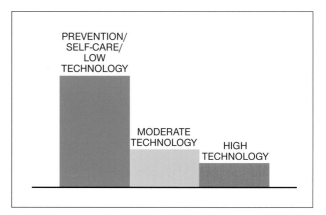

Fig 14 Eventual future distribution of tasks in oral health care in all countries. (Modified from WHO, 1994. Reprinted with permission.)

18

cently developed chemicals are used to soften and disclose the carious dentin in the cavity. For small carious cavities, hand instruments can be used to scrape out the diseased tissue. The damaged area can be repaired with glass-ionomer cement, which also has a preventive effect, functioning as a slow-releasing fluoride agent that can be recharged with fluoride from other agents, such as fluoride toothpaste. The aim of the first level (low technology) of oral care is to prevent the need for more traditional and costly invasive (moderate technology) oral care.

The second level (moderate technology) includes multiple-surface restorations, extractions, simple periodontal surgery, and removable prostheses—that is, traditional invasive oral care, practiced by most dentists worldwide.

The third and most complex, high-technology level of oral care includes precision prosthetics; implants; laminates and ceramic inlays and onlays; orthodontics; regenerative periodontal treatment; and complex oral surgery and medicine—in other words, costly and complex procedures that require highly qualified specialists or "oral physicians." Therefore, in any society, the availability of high-technology oral care will be limited.

A rational, health-promoting, affordable mix of oral care should be planned and implemented in all countries. Emphasis on prevention and control of oral diseases will minimize the need for intervention at the moderate- and high-technology levels. As a consequence of improving oral health in most industrialized countries, the need for moderately complex care is decreasing. With further emphasis on prevention, the need and demand for first-level interventions will increase slightly, while the need for high-technology care will probably increase for several decades, because of the desire to preserve natural teeth and the increasing numbers of elderly people who have some natural teeth and edentulous people who want implant treatment.

In developing countries, the first (low-technology, noninvasive) level of oral care will continue to be the major need. In those developing countries where the prevalence of caries is increasing, a rising demand for moderate-technology care will continue over the next few decades. High-technology oral care must, on the other hand, still be limited.

The proportion of the population taking advantage of oral health care services varies from country to country, but in only a few might it be considered optimum. For example, in Sweden, almost 100% of 1 to 19 year olds receive well-organized and regular oral care, predominantly preventive dentistry, free of charge (Axelsson et al, 1993a). In the county of Värmland, Sweden, 95% of the adult population visits oral health care clinics regularly for oral care, including prevention (Axelsson and Paulander, 1994). In most countries, total coverage is an unrealistic goal, but steps should be taken to ensure that oral care is available to all those who need it.

The pattern of oral health care levels in highly industrialized countries, from the past to the future, is shown in Figs 10 to 12, modified from the WHO (WHO's Oral Health Unit Data Bank, 1994).

The typical distribution and trends of different oral health care levels in developing countries are shown in Fig 13. The eventual future distribution of oral health care levels in all countries is illustrated in Fig 14.

CHAPTER 3

ETIOLOGIC FACTORS IN ORAL DISEASES

PLAQUE

Colonization of the tooth surfaces by bacteria is acknowledged as the key etiologic factor in the most common oral diseases—dental caries, gingivitis, and the destructive periodontal diseases. As long ago as 1954, Orland et al demonstrated that germ-free animals do not develop caries. Furthermore, in humans, when bacteria are allowed to accumulate in plaque on the tooth surfaces, enamel caries and gingivitis develop within 2 or 3 weeks (Löe et al, 1965; Theilade et al, 1966; Von der Fehr et al, 1970).

Like the inflammation induced in the gingival soft tissues adjacent to the gingival plaque, carious lesions of enamel, which develop on individual tooth surfaces beneath the bacterial plaque, represent the net result of an extraordinarily complex interplay among "harmless" and "harmful" bacteria, antagonistic and synergistic bacterial species, their metabolic products, and their interaction with the many salivary and other host factors. This explains why combinations of different nonspecific plaque control programs have been so effective against caries and gingivitis as well as periodontitis (for reviews see Axelsson, 1994, 1998).

Plaque formation

According to Dawes et al (1963), dental plaque is "the soft tenacious material found on tooth surfaces which is not readily removed by rinsing with water." It is estimated that 1 mm^3 of dental plaque, weighing about 1 mg, will contain more than 200 million bacteria (Scheie, 1994). Other microorganisms, such as mycoplasma, yeasts, and protozoa, also occur in mature plaque; sticky polysaccharides and other products form the so-called plaque matrix, which comprises 10% to 40% by volume of the supragingival plaque (Scheie, 1994).

The most readily discernible plaque, on the smooth surfaces of the teeth, along the gingival margin, is termed *dentogingival plaque*. Dentogingival plaque on the approximal surfaces, apical to the contact points, is termed *approximal dental plaque*. Plaque occurring below the gingival margin, in the gingival sulcus or in the periodontal pocket, is termed *subgingival plaque* (Theilade and Theilade, 1976).

Although there are well over 350 species of bacteria in the oral cavity, only a few have the ability to colonize a newly cleaned tooth surface. This initial association depends on the presentation and interaction of surface molecules on the bacteria and the pellicle-coated tooth surface. The ini-

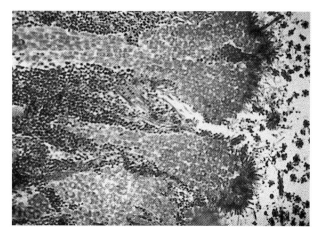

Fig 15 Cross section of columns of colonizing bacteria, separated by open spaces. (From Listgarten, 1975. Reprinted with permission.)

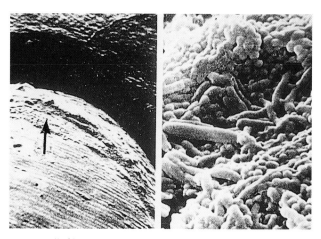

Fig 16 (left) Scanning electron micrograph of plaque formation along the gingival margin (arrow) after 24 to 48 hours. (right) Increased magnification revealing that the plaque is dominated by streptococci and a few rods. (From Saxton, 1975. Reprinted with permission.)

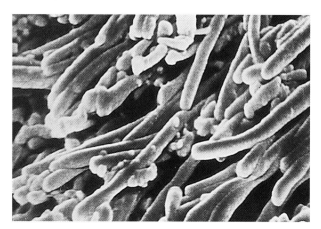

Fig 17 Outer surface of plaque in phase II of plaque development, covered by gram-positive tall rods. (From Saxton, 1975. Reprinted with permission.)

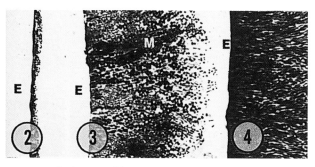

Fig 18 Thickness of freely accumulated gingival plaque after 2, 3, and 4 days. E = tooth enamel; M = microbial plaque. (From Listgarten, 1975. Reprinted with permission.)

Fig 19 Cross section of gingival plaque filling the gingival sulcus while spirochetes and vibrios move around in the outer and more apical regions of the sulcus. (From Listgarten, 1976. Reprinted with permission.)

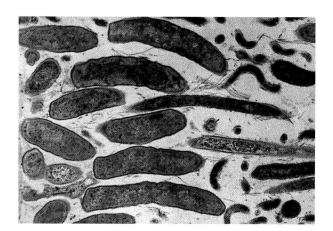

Fig 20 Diseased periodontal pocket containing attached sub-gingival plaque and nonattaching, motile subgingival microflora (spirochetes, vibrios, and straight rods with flagella).

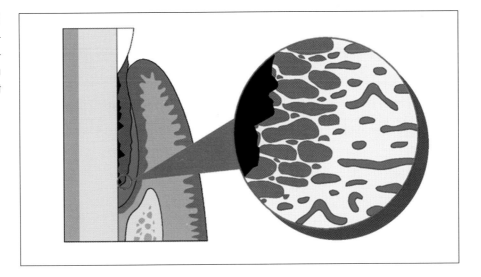

tial bacteria are called *pioneer colonizers*, because they are hardy and successfully compete with other members of the oral flora for a place on the tooth surface. After initial deposition, clones of pioneer colonizing bacteria begin to expand away from the tooth surface to form columns that move outward in long chains of pallisading bacteria. These parallel columns of bacteria are separated by uniformly narrow spaces (Fig 15). Plaque growth proceeds by deposition of new species into these open spaces.

Within a short time, the tooth surface adjacent to the gingiva is covered by intermeshed bacteria. New bacteria derived from saliva or surrounding mucous membranes now sense only the bacteria-laden landscape of the tooth surface and attach by a bonding interaction to bacteria already attached to the plaque. All this activity occurs within the first 2 days of plaque development and, for descriptive purposes, is called *phase I* of plaque formation. As shown in Fig 16, continuous plaque has formed along the gingival margin after 24 to 48 hours. A close-up confirms that the plaque is dominated by streptococci and a few rods.

In *phase II* of plaque development, the outer surface of the plaque is covered by gram-positive tall rods (Fig 17). Figure 18 illustrates the thickness of freely accumulated gingival plaque after 2, 3, and 4 days. There is a dramatic increase in plaque thickness after 3 and 4 days compared to the first 2 days.

In *phase III*, 4 to 7 days after initiation, plaque begins to migrate subgingivally, and bacteria and their products permeate and circulate in the pocket. In *phase IV*, 7 to 11 days after initiation of plaque development, the diversity of the flora increases to comprise motile bacteria including spirochetes and vibrios as well as fusiforms. Figure 19 shows, in cross section, how attached gingival plaque fills the gingival sulcus while spirochetes and vibrios move around in the outer and more apical regions of the sulcus.

This mature plaque is now so packed with diverse bacteria that an exogenous species would have great difficulty becoming established in the overcrowded habitat. With time, more bacteria migrate subgingivally, and the process continues more aggressively. The critical locus of activity is the subgingival space (periodontal pocket). The bacteria residing in the pocket and the host cells that defend it determine the clinical outcome. The diseased periodontal pocket harbors both attached subgingival plaque biofilms and nonattaching, motile subgingival microflora (spirochetes, vibrios, and straight rods with flagella) (Fig 20).

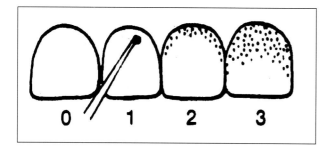

Fig 21 Silness and Löe Plaque Index (1965): 0 = the tooth surface is clean; 1 = the tooth surface appears clean, but dental plaque can be removed from the gingival third with a sharp explorer; 2 = visible plaque is present along the gingival margin; 3 = the tooth surface is covered with abundant plaque.

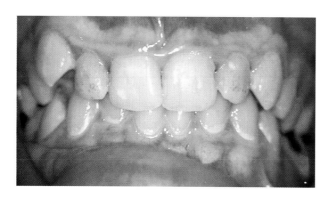

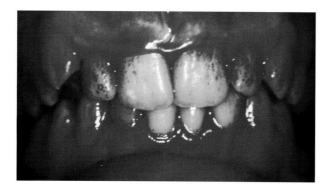

Fig 22 Anterior teeth of a 12-year-old boy with gingivitis at the following sites: the mesiobuccal (MB) surface of tooth 13; the MB surface of tooth 12; the distobuccal (DB) surface of tooth 21; the MB and DB surfaces of tooth 22; the MB surface of tooth 23; the MB surface of tooth 43; the DB surface of tooth 42; the DB surface of tooth 32; and the MB surface of tooth 33. Enamel (incipient) caries is located at the MB surface of tooth 13; the MB surface of tooth 43; the buccal surface of tooth 42; the DB surface of tooth 32; the MB surface of tooth 33; and the MB surface of tooth 34. In addition, a cavity is present on the distal surface of tooth 22.

Fig 23 Erythosin-stained dentition of the patient in Fig 22. Note the close correspondence between areas of plaque and areas affected by gingivitis and caries.

Plaque indices

Several indices have been developed for recording supragingival plaque. The two most frequently used are the Plaque Index developed by Silness and Löe (1964) and O'Leary's Plaque Index (O'Leary et al, 1972).

The Silness and Löe Plaque Index has a four-point scale (Fig 21): Score 0 = the tooth surface is clean; score 1 = the tooth surface appears clean, but dental plaque can be removed from the gingival third with a sharp explorer; score 2 = visible plaque is present along the gingival margin; and score 3 = the tooth surface is covered with abundant plaque.

O'Leary's Plaque Index is based on the presence or absence of visible continuous plaque along the gingival margin after staining. The percentage of tooth surfaces exhibiting stained plaque is calculated. Four or six surfaces per tooth are diagnosed. Unlike Silness and Löe's Plaque Index, no attempts are made to evaluate the area of tooth surface covered by plaque.

O'Leary's Plaque Index is most commonly used for evaluation of the oral hygiene standard of the individual patient and for patient motivation, based on self-diagnosis. However, use of O'Leary's Plaque Index in dental practice reveals only the number of areas that the patient has failed to clean effectively even though he or she made a special effort on the day of the dental appointment. It does not indicate the rate at which plaque forms in the individual or the patient's oral hygiene status 1 week before or after the dental appointment.

Despite these limitations, the staining of plaque is the fastest and most efficient means to allow self-diagnosis by the patient and to allow the clinician to locate remaining plaque and to visualize the close relationship between the location of plaque and the existence of gingivitis and dental caries. This principle is illustrated in Figs 22 and 23. Figure 22 shows the anterior teeth of a 12-year-old boy with gingivitis and enamel (incipient) caries. Because the dental plaque was semitranslucent, it was visualized by using a disclosing (erythrosin) pellet (Fig 23). There is a close relationship between the location of the stained plaque shown in Fig 23 and the location of gingivitis and dental caries shown in Fig 22. Therefore, prevention of dental caries and gingivitis must be based on plaque control.

Plaque formation rate and pattern

The quantity of plaque that forms on clean tooth surfaces during a given time represents the net result of interactions among etiologic factors, many internal and external risk indicators and risk factors, as well as protective factors:

1. The total oral bacterial population
2. The quality of the oral bacterial flora
3. The anatomy and surface morphology of the dentition
4. The wettability and surface tension of the tooth surfaces
5. The salivary secretion rate and other properties of saliva
6. The intake of fermentable carbohydrates
7. The mobility of the tongue and lips
8. The exposure to chewing forces and abrasion from foods
9. The degree of gingival inflammation and volume of gingival exudate
10. The individual oral hygiene habits
11. The use of fluorides and other preventive products, such as chemical plaque control agents

This observation has been the rationale for the construction of the Plaque Formation Rate Index (PFRI) (Axelsson, 1987, 1991). It includes all but the occlusal tooth surfaces and is based on the amount of plaque freely accumulated in the 24 hours after professional mechanical tooth cleaning, during which period the subjects refrain from all oral hygiene. In a pilot study on 50 adult subjects, adherent plaque was disclosed on 5% to 65% of the total number of tooth surfaces (Axelsson, 1983). On the basis of this study, the following five-point scale was constructed for the PFRI:

score 1 = 1% to 10% of surfaces affected: very low
score 2 = 11% to 20% of surfaces affected: low
score 3 = 21% to 30% of surfaces affected: moderate
score 4 = 31% to 40% of surfaces affected: high
score 5 = ≥ 41% of surfaces affected: very high

Figure 24 shows the frequency distribution of PFRI scores 1 to 5 among 667 14-year-old children in the city of Karlstad, Sweden, where the standard of oral hygiene is very high and caries prevalence is very low (Axelsson, 1987, 1991). The majority of children were low (score 2 = 48%) or moderate (score 3 = 27%) plaque formers.

In contrast, studies in Brazil (Axelsson et al,

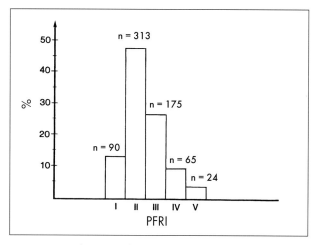

Fig 24 Stratification of plaque formation rate index (PFRI) in 14 year olds in Karlstad, Sweden. (From Axelsson, 1991. Reprinted with permission.)

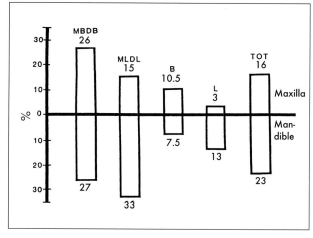

Fig 25 Plaque formation rate in 14-year-old subjects 24 hours after professional mechanical tooth cleaning. (MB) mesiobuccal; (DB) distobuccal; (ML) mesiolingual; (DL) distolingual; (B) buccal; (L) lingual; (TOT) total. (From Axelsson, 1991. Reprinted with permission.)

1994), Germany (Cunea and Axelsson, 1997), and Poland (Axelsson et al, 1999a), where caries prevalence is high to very high, have revealed that the majority of 12- to 15-year-old children are high to very high plaque formers (PFRI scores 4 and 5). In addition, young subjects with high PFRI scores develop more gingivitis than do those with low scores (Axelsson, 1987; Ramberg et al, 1995a). There is also a strong correlation between plaque formation rate and gingivitis at the surface level (Ramberg et al, 1995a).

For successful strategies for primary as well as secondary prevention of dental caries and periodontal disease, an understanding of plaque formation rates and patterns is extremely important. There is overwhelming evidence indicating that complete mechanical removal of bacterial plaque from the dentogingival region is the most effective method of preventing gingivitis and periodontitis, further supporting the nonspecific plaque hypothesis (Lövdahl et al, 1961; Axelsson and Lindhe, 1974, 1977, 1978; Axelsson et al, 1991, 1994; for reviews, see Axelsson 1981, 1993, 1994, 1998; Kieser, 1994).

As discussed earlier, the plaque formation rate is influenced by such factors as the anatomy and

surface morphology of the teeth, the stage of eruption and functional status of the teeth, the wettability and surface tension of the tooth surfaces (both intact and restored surfaces), and the gingival health and volume of gingival exudate. The pattern of plaque reaccumulation will also be influenced by the same factors but may differ somewhat on tooth surfaces exposed to chewing forces; abrasion from foods; and friction from the dorsum of the tongue, lips, and cheeks; and on less accessible areas, such as approximal sites, along the gingival margin, and in irregularities such as occlusal fissures. These areas are often designated *stagnation areas* for plaque. Figure 25 presents the percentage of freely reaccumulated (de novo) plaque 24 hours after professional mechanical tooth cleaning on the surfaces of maxillary and mandibular teeth from the large-scale study of 667 14 year olds in the city of Karlstad, Sweden (Axelsson, 1987, 1991). Plaque reaccumulation was greatest on the mandibular mesiolingual and distolingual surfaces (33%), particularly on the molars, followed by the mesiobuccal and distobuccal surfaces on both maxillary and mandibular teeth, particularly the molars. There was almost no plaque reaccumulation (3%) on the

Fig 26 Reaccumulation of plaque (shaded areas) at 48 hours in partially and fully erupted molars. (Modified from Carvalho et al, 1989.)

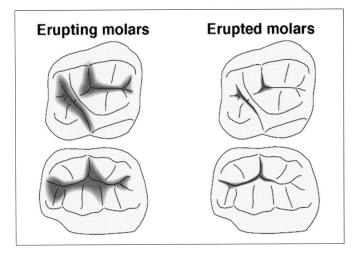

lingual surfaces of the maxillary teeth, mainly because of friction from the rough dorsum of the tongue. It should be noted that the pattern of dental caries and gingivitis in young adults is almost identical to the pattern of plaque reaccumulation.

Carvallo et al (1989) studied the pattern and amount of de novo plaque, 48 hours after professional mechanical tooth cleaning, on the occlusal surfaces of partially and fully erupted first molars. Figure 26 illustrates the heavy plaque reaccumulation found, particularly in the distal and central fossae, in the erupting maxillary and mandibular molars, in contrast to the reaccumulation in fully erupted molars, subjected to normal chewing friction. Abrasion from normal mastication significantly limits plaque formation. This explains why almost 100% of occlusal caries in molars begins in the distal and central fossae during the eruption period of 14 to 18 months (Carvalho et al, 1989).

Plaque ecology

The ecological plaque hypothesis is based on the theory that the unique local microenvironment influences the composition of the oral microflora (Marsh, 1994). From an ecological point of view, the oral cavity is an open growth system; that is, nutrients and microbes are repeatedly introduced to and removed from the system. The flow rate of saliva is so high that, to colonize the surfaces of the oral cavity, the organisms must be able to adhere or be retained in some other way. Not only the flow of saliva but also the flow of the gingival fluid, chewing, oral hygiene procedures, and desquamation of epithelial cells from the mucous membranes serve to remove bacteria from the oral surfaces. Some bacteria may remain simply by obtaining a refuge in pits and fissures or in the protected areas between the teeth. Other microorganisms have to rely on specific mechanisms of adherence to overcome the strong removal forces on the oral surfaces.

The characteristics of the oral surfaces are unique, and only specific bacteria have the ability to adhere. This means that the oral cavity harbors a unique microbiota, and most species are unable to colonize any other site of the human body. The oral cavity consists of several distinct sites, each of which will support the growth of a characteristic microbial community. Enormous differences thus exist in the composition of the microbiota on the mucous membranes, the tongue, the teeth and in the gingival sulcus area. It has even been demonstrated that the composition of the microbiota may vary from site to site on a single tooth surface (Marsh, 1989). For example, facultative anaerobes able to attach to the solid tooth surfaces predominate in thin supragingival plaque on buccal and lingual surfaces, while obligate anaerobic spirochetes predominate at the base of deep periodontal pockets.

Similarly, low pH and access to fermentable carbohydrates such as sucrose provide a favorable environment for aciduric and acidogenic bacteria (eg, *Streptococcus mutans* and *lactobacilli*). Dental practitioners spend most of their clinical time dealing with problems caused by the oral microflora and emphasize improved methods of removing or inhibiting this source of inflammation and disease. However, the normal oral microflora is an important defense factor, acting in concert with other host defenses to help prevent colonization by exogenous, and often pathogenic, microorganisms.

Nevertheless, occasionally, imbalances in the stability of the resident oral microflora do occur and predispose a site to disease. This may arise because of changes in diet, hormones, the use of antimicrobial agents, deficiencies in the host defenses, or inadequate plaque control. Therefore, during the treatment and management of patients, the aim of the dentist should be to identify any predisposing factors and select strategies to control rather than eliminate, the oral microflora, so as to preserve the beneficial properties of the harmless normal oral microflora.

PATHOGENIC BACTERIA

Both dental caries and the periodontal diseases are infectious and transmissible diseases; that is, exogenous pathogenic bacteria related to the etiology of these diseases can be transmitted from one individual to another, mostly from mouth to mouth within families. However, there are also endogenous presumptive pathogens, which may result in opportunistic infections under special conditions.

Specific microflora related to the etiology of dental caries

Mutans streptococci (MS) have been shown to be an exogenous and transmissible cariogenic group of bacteria in animal experiments as well as in human studies (Keyes, 1960; Köhler and Bratthall, 1978). For example, it was shown that babies were infected by MS from mothers with high salivary levels of MS as soon as the first primary teeth erupted (Köhler and Bratthall, 1978). Mutans streptococci are acidogenic and aciduric, can produce extracellular polysaccharides, and adhere to tooth surfaces. In other words, MS have all the requirements for a caries-inducing group of bacteria, a fact that has been confirmed in numerous human and animal studies (see Bratthall, 1991; Bowden, 1991; and Bratthall and Ericsson, 1994, for reviews).

In populations with a high caries prevalence, there is a correlation between salivary MS levels and both caries prevalence and caries incidence. Mutans streptococci counts greater than 1 million per milliliter of saliva are considered to indicate a high caries risk (Klock and Krasse, 1979; Zickert et al, 1982). However, in populations with low caries prevalence, the threshold for caries risk seems to be whether the individual is MS negative or MS positive, so that the 15% to 25% of the population that is MS negative should be regarded as being without caries risk. Among the 75% to 80% of the population that is MS positive, low-risk, moderate-risk, and high-risk individuals should be selected in relation to the plaque formation rate (Axelsson, 1987, 1991) (Fig 27).

However, there is undoubtedly a strong correlation between the number of MS in dental plaque at the tooth surface and the risk of development of enamel caries. It was found, in a 30-month investigation, that a continuously high number of MS on the approximal tooth surfaces resulted in caries on about 70% of these surfaces. On the other hand, of all the surfaces with little or no MS, only one was carious (Axelsson et al, 1987b). An earlier study found that the highest

Fig 27 Four-point scale for prediction of caries risk, based on the amount of mutans streptococci (MS) per milliliter (mL) of saliva and the Plaque Formation Rate Index (PRFI). (Modified from Axelsson, 1991.)

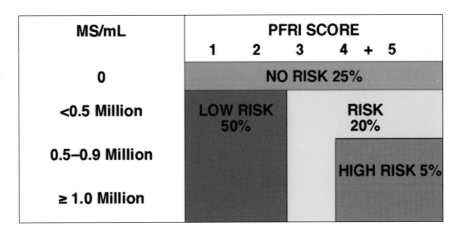

MS/mL	PFRI SCORE			
	1	2	3	4 + 5
0	NO RISK 25%			
<0.5 Million	LOW RISK 50%		RISK 20%	
0.5–0.9 Million				
≥ 1.0 Million			HIGH RISK 5%	

Fig 28 In members of toothbrushing populations, dental caries is concentrated in the approximal surfaces of the posterior teeth. Therefore, supplementary plaque control methods should be performed on these high-risk surfaces. (From Waerhaug, 1981. Reprinted with permission of the University of Oslo.)

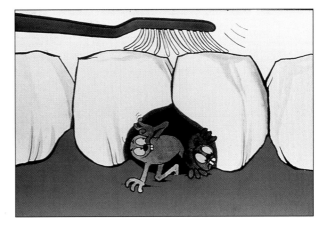

numbers of MS were located on the approximal surfaces of the molars and the second premolars (Kristoffersson et al, 1984). Therefore, for plaque prevention in a toothbrushing population, plaque control and topical fluorides should be directed toward these key-risk surfaces: approximal surfaces of the molars and premolars (Fig 28).

There are more acidogenic and aciduric bacteria among the normal oral microflora, and these should be regarded as cariogenic bacteria under special conditions, such as low pH and high intake of sucrose; that is, they are opportunistic caries-inducing bacteria. Among these are groups of lactobacilli, actinomyces, and *Streptococcus salivarius*. Mutans streptococci are associated with fissure caries and smooth-surface caries as well as root caries, while groups of lactobacilli are associated with fissure caries, deep dentinal carious lesions, and root caries. Both *S salivarius* and groups of actinomyces are associated with fissure caries, deep dentinal carious lesions, and root caries.

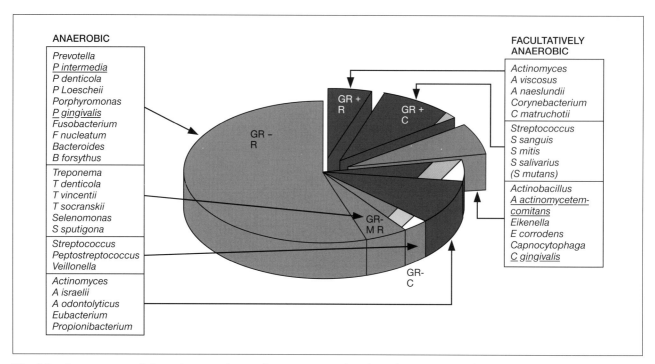

Fig 29 Composition of the subgingival microflora associated with early-onset periodontitis. The most important periopathogens are underlined. GR+ = gram-positive microorganisms (blue); GR– = gram-negative microorganisms (red); R = rod-shaped microorganisms; C = cocci-shaped microorganisms; MR = motile rod-shaped microorganisms.

Specific microflora related to the etiology of periodontal diseases

Marginal periodontal diseases are infectious diseases, which may be categorized as early-onset periodontitis (localized or generalized), acute necrotizing (ulcerative) periodontitis, or adult marginal periodontitis. Figures 29 to 31 show the estimated composition of the subgingival microflora associated with these three categories of periodontal disease; the most important periopathogens are underlined. *Actinobacillus actinomycetemcomitans* and *Porphyromonas gingivalis* are regarded as exogenous, transmissible periopathogens, resulting in true infection, while others, such as *Bacteroides forsythus, Prevotella intermedia, Eikenella corrodens,* and different spirochetes, represent endogenous infection. In the compromised host, such microorganisms will result in opportunistic infection (van Winkelhoff et al, 1996).

For many years, it has been suggested that the mode of infection is transmission of periodontal pathogens by direct contact (Alaluusua et al, 1991). The putative periodontal pathogens are obligate and facultative anaerobic bacteria, with no known ecological niche other than the oral cavity. Viable forms of these organisms are found in saliva, and there is evidence of direct transmission within families. Other sites in the oral cavity should therefore be considered as potential reservoirs of periodontopathogens, capable of infecting periodontal sites in susceptible individuals. Both *A actinomycetemcomitans* and *P gingivalis* can be transmitted from patients with periodontal disease to family members (Zambon et al, 1983; Alaluusua et al, 1991; Preus et al, 1994; Petit et al, 1993a, 1993b, 1994; van Steenbergen et al, 1993). Microbial testing of spouses and children in families with members who are affected by periodontitis may determine possible transmission of pathogens and form the basis for early disease intervention in susceptible individuals (Saarela et al, 1993; von Troil-Linden et al, 1995).

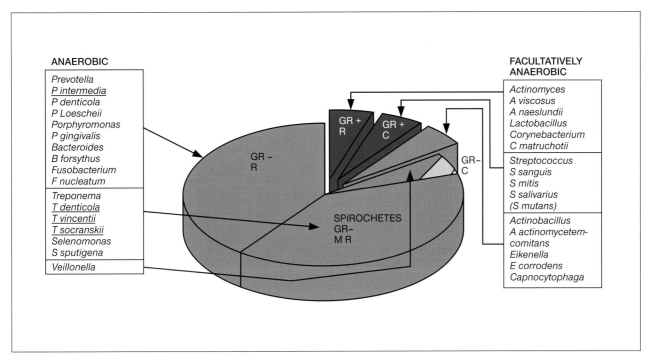

Fig 30 Composition of the subgingival microflora associated with acute necrotizing (ulcerative) periodontitis. The most important periopathogens are underlined. GR+ = gram-positive microorganisms (blue); GR− = gram-negative microorganisms (red); R = rod-shaped microorganisms; C = cocci-shaped microorganisms; MR = motile rod-shaped microorganisms.

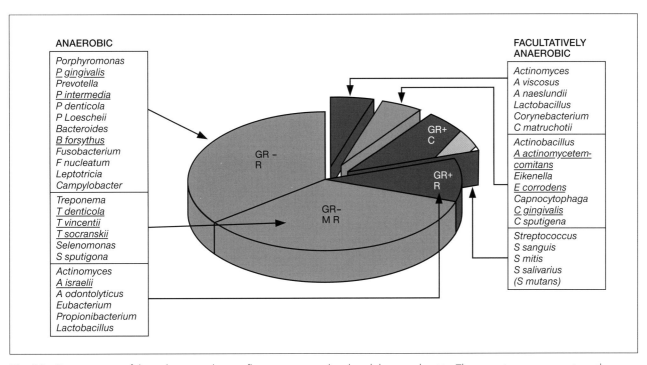

Fig 31 Composition of the subgingival microflora associated with adult periodontitis. The most important periopathogens are underlined. GR+ = gram-positive microorganisms (blue); GR− = gram-negative microorganisms (red); R = rod-shaped microorganisms; C = cocci-shaped microorganisms; MR = motile rod-shaped microorganisms.

Actinobacillus actinomycetemcomitans, P intermedia, and *E corrodens* seem to be associated with early-onset periodontitis (see Fig 29). Acute necrotizing ulcerative periodontitis is caused by a superinfection of particularly *P intermedia* and spirochetes such as *Treponema denticola* and *Treponema vincentii* (see Fig 30). The predominating periopathogens associated with adult periodontitis are *P gingivalis, B forsythus, P intermedia,* and *T denticola* (see Fig 31). In a recent study, it was shown that there was a seventimes increased risk for further loss of periodontal attachment at sites infected by *Bacteroides forsythus* (Machtei et al, 1997). It was recently shown that this bacteria occurs more frequently in diseased periodontal pockets in smokers than in nonsmokers (Zambon et al, 1996a).

CHAPTER 4

MODIFYING FACTORS IN ORAL DISEASES

DEFINITION OF TERMS

Besides etiologic, preventive, and control factors, many other factors may modify the prevalence, onset, and progression of dental caries and periodontal diseases. Such factors are divided into external (environmental) and internal (endogenous) factors.

Factors that have proved to be significantly associated with increased prevalence of a specific disease in cross-sectional studies are termed *risk indicators* (RIs). Factors that have proved to significantly increase the risk for onset and/or progression of a specific disease in well-controlled prospective studies are termed *risk factors* (RFs) and *prognostic risk factors* (PRFs), respectively. The RFs and PRFs are often expressed in *odds ratio* (OR) for onset or progression of a specific disease.

EXTERNAL (ENVIRONMENTAL) RISK INDICATORS, RISK FACTORS, AND PROGNOSTIC RISK FACTORS

Dental caries

Among external modifying RIs, RFs, and PRFs for dental caries are fermentable carbohydrates (particularly high frequency of sugar intake), poor socioeconomic conditions, systemic diseases, medicines with salivary depressive effects, and irregular dental care habits.

In the classic 5-year prospective Vipeholm study from Sweden (Gustavsson et al, 1954), it was shown that caries incidence is correlated with the frequency of intake of sugar-containing products. In other words, extended sugar clearance time is an external modifying risk factor or prognostic risk factor for caries development. However, the study was carried out under extreme conditions: test subjects were mentally handicapped people with heavy amounts of plaque and no oral hygiene. In the most extreme group, 24 large, sticky, sugar-containing toffees per day were distributed between meals. In spite of this extreme challenge, about 30% of this group did not develop any carious lesions during the 5-year period.

On the other hand, if the standard of oral hygiene is very high, even a high frequency of sugar intake will fail to increase development of caries. In the absence of oral hygiene, dental students who rinsed nine times per day with a 50% sucrose solution developed enamel smooth-surface lesions within 3 weeks (von der Fehr et al, 1970). However, another group of dental students, who rinsed twice per day with 0.2% chlorhexidine solution (chemical plaque control), did not develop enamel caries despite rinsing with a 50% sucrose solution nine times per day (Löe et al, 1972). It has also been shown that germ-free animals do not develop caries despite frequent sugar intake (Orland et al, 1954); when they are infected by cariogenic bacteria, however, they develop rampant caries (Keyes, 1960).

The conclusions drawn from these studies are (*1*) "clean teeth never decay"; and (*2*) sugar is not an etiologic but an external modifying risk factor. However, its power is very weak in populations with low caries prevalence, high standards of oral hygiene, and daily use of fluoride toothpaste (Kristoffersson et al, 1986). On the other hand, in populations with poor oral hygiene, no use of fluoride toothpaste, and relatively high caries prevalence, frequent intake of sugar (prolonged sugar clearance time) should still be regarded as a powerful external modifying risk factor.

Among socioeconomic factors, low educational level seems to be an important external modifying risk indicator and risk factor (Axelsson et al, 1990; Paulander et al, 1999). A high percentage of the most commonly prescribed medicines, such as psychopharmaceuticals and antihistamines, have a very significant depressive effect on salivary secretion rate and should therefore be regarded as external modifying RIs, RFs, and PRFs for dental caries (Axelsson et al, 1990).

Periodontal diseases

Examples of external modifying RIs, RFs, and PRFs for periodontal diseases are smoking, use of smokeless tobacco, irregular dental care, low socioeconomic level, infectious and other acquired diseases, side effects of medication, and poor dietary habits. Among these, smoking and irregular dental care habits are the most important and common.

Numerous cross-sectional studies have shown that smoking is a very powerful external modifying RI for periodontal diseases. In a multifactorial analytical study, smoking was ranked number 1 (after age) as a risk indicator for periodontal attachment loss (Grossi et al, 1994). Among 65 year olds, it was estimated that smokers had lost about 50% more periodontal attachment than nonsmokers when calculations were adjusted for the greater number of lost teeth in the former group (Axelsson et al, 1998; for review, see Bergström and Preber, 1994; Axelsson et al, 1998).

In a recent prospective study, it was shown that the risk for further progression of periodontal disease was about five times higher in smokers than in nonsmokers (Machtei et al, 1997). It has also been shown that the outcome of periodontal therapy, including regenerative therapy, is significantly impaired in smokers compared to nonsmokers (Ah et al, 1994; Tonetti et al, 1995). In other words, smoking is an extremely powerful external modifying risk factor as well as prognostic risk factor for periodontal onset and progression.

In a randomized sample of more than 600 50 to 55 year olds, it was shown that subjects with irregular dental care habits had lost almost 50% more periodontal attachment than had subjects with regular dental care habits (Axelsson and Paulander, 1994). Other cross-sectional studies have also shown that adult subjects (35, 50, 65, and 75 year olds) with low educational level have lost more periodontal attachment than have subjects with higher educational level (Axelsson et al, 1990; Paulander et al, 1999).

Some infectious and acquired diseases, especially severe diseases, such as ulcerous colitis, Crohn's disease, acquired immunodeficiency syndrome, and leukemia, will also be strong risk factors and prognostic risk factors for periodontal diseases. However, the opposite may also apply: In a recently published 18-year longitudinal study, a direct linear correlation was shown among the number of diseased periodontal pockets, the amount of lost periodontal support, and the risk for development of cardiovascular disease and stroke (Beck et al, 1996). This may be explained in part by the effects of endotoxins from the gram-negative, subgingival microflora on the endothelial cells of the blood vessels. The risk for development of cardiovascular disease and stroke was correlated somewhat higher with periodontal disease than with smoking but slightly less than with hereditary factors (for review, see Beck et al, 1996).

INTERNAL (ENDOGENOUS) RISK INDICATORS, RISK FACTORS, AND PROGNOSTIC RISK FACTORS

Dental caries

Internal RIs, RFs, and PFRs for dental caries are reduced salivary secretion rate, reduced quality of the saliva, impaired host factors, chronic diseases, unfavorable macroanatomy and microanatomy of the teeth that favor plaque retention, and poor quality of enamel or dentin. Reduced salivary secretion rate seems to be the most important. Normal, low, and hyposalivation values for unstimulated and stimulated whole saliva are shown in Table 3.

Analytical epidemiologic studies have shown that about 15%, 20%, and 25% in randomized samples of 50-, 65-, and 75-year-old subjects, respectively, had less than 0.70 mL of stimulated salivary

secretion per minute. In addition there was a strong correlation between salivary secretion rate and caries prevalence (Axelsson et al, 1990).

There are exogenous as well as endogenous causes of hyposalivation. By far the most common exogenous reason is medication, followed by irradiation to the head and neck area. The main endogenous causes are chronic diseases (rheumatoid arthritis, Sjögren´s syndrome, and labile type I diabetes mellitus), menopause, anorexia nervosa, and malnutrition (dehydration).

Although saliva has several functions, the most important one is the clearance of oral microorganisms and food components from the oral cavity to the gut. Therefore, an adequate volume of saliva to flush pathogenic (and also commensal) microorganisms from the oral cavity is a requirement for a healthy balance between host defense and endogenous and exogenous microbial attack in the mouth.

The plaque formation rate is influenced by the volume as well as the quality of saliva. From a caries risk aspect, poor buffer capacity and inadequate fluoride concentration seem to be the most important quality factors. However, the combined effects of insufficient levels of secretory immunoglobulin A against cariogenic bacteria, antimicrobial enzymes, agglutinins, inorganic calcium, and phosphates may also have some importance.

In addition, the volume of gingival exudate, and the macroanatomy and microanatomy and eruption stage of the teeth will influence the plaque formation rate, as well as the pattern of plaque formation and mutans streptococci in the dentition.

Table 3 Salivary secretion rates (mL/min)				
Whole saliva	(mean)	Normal (range)	Low (range)	Hyposalivation
Unstimulated	0.30	0.25 – 0.35	0.10 – 0.25	< 0.10
Paraffin-stimulated	2.00	1.00 – 3.00	0.70 – 1.00	< 0.70

Periodontal diseases

Internal RIs, RFs, and PRFs related to periodontal diseases are genetic factors, impaired host factors, chronic diseases, and reduced salivary flow and quality.

Most studies of genetic factors in periodontal disease have examined the early-onset forms of disease, ie, prepubertal, juvenile (localized and generalized), and rapidly progressive periodontitis, on the grounds that, compared to the adult chronic form, aggressive disease in young individuals is less likely to result from chronic environmental (bacterial plaque) insults (Michalowicz et al, 1991a, 1991b; Michalowicz, 1994a. Furthermore, patients with early-onset disease probably represent a more homogenous population than do those with chronic adult periodontitis (Michalowicz, 1994a).

Studies of families suggest that susceptibility to the early-onset forms of disease, particularly prepubertal and juvenile periodontitis, is at least in part influenced by host genotype. Inherited phagocytic cell deficiencies appear to confer risk for prepubertal periodontitis. The prevalence and distribution of early-onset periodontitis in affected families are most consistent with an autosomal-recessive mode of inheritance.

Comparisons between adult monozygotic twins reared together and reared apart indicate that early family environment has no appreciable influence on probing depth and attachment loss measures in adults. In the Minnesota twin periodontal study (Michalowicz et al, 1991a, 1991b), it was calculated that, among 38% to 82% of the population, variance of attachment loss, probing depth, and Gingival Index may be attributed to genetic factors in monozygotic and dizygotic adult twins, both reared together and reared apart.

Updated and additional data from this study show that genetic factors not only contribute to the overall extent of disease but also may influence the distribution or pattern of disease. To examine the specific influence of genetic factors on disease, the odds were computed of one twin having disease at a specific site or tooth if the cotwin had disease at the site. For both twin groups, reared together and reared apart, the odds ratios were greater for monozygotic than dizygotic twins (Michalowicz, 1994a).

The Virginia twin study, based on self-reported periodontal disease in an adult population, also confirmed that periodontal disease in monozygotic twins is significantly more concordant than in dizygotic twins (Corey et al, 1993).

A number of apparently genetically determined syndromes or diseases appear to carry an associated increased risk for periodontal destruction. In a few cases, there appears to be a defect that predisposes the carrier to destruction of the periodontal tissues because the absence of, or abnormal regulation of, a tissue component necessary for structural integrity, such as the collagen defect of Ehlers-Danlos syndrome and possibly insulin-dependent juvenile diabetes. In other syndromes or diseases, defects of phagocytic cell function have been described, especially polymorphonuclear leukocytes (PMNLs), but also mononuclear phagocytes. In diseases such as juvenile diabetes, these phagocytic defects are found in the presence of possible disorders of collagen regulation, such as excess production of collagenase in the gingiva. Although there are more data on PMNL dysfunction, it is possible that further studies will also reveal defects of mononuclear phagocytes associated with these syndromes.

Recently, Kornman et al (1997) reported a specific genotype of the polymorphic interleukin-1 gene cluster that was associated with severity of periodontitis in nonsmokers and distinguished individuals with severe periodontitis from those with mild periodontitis (odds ratio 18.9 for persons aged 40 to 60 years). It is estimated that almost 30% of the adult population exhibits this genotype of interleukin-1. Based on these findings, the Periodontal Susceptibility Test was developed.

Studies of host response in periodontal diseases have clearly indicated the polymorphonuclear leukocyte (neutrophil PMNL) as the key protective cell that, under normal circumstances, limits the pathosis caused by periodontal organisms. The PMNL does not act alone and operates as part of a PMNL-antibody-complement axis that exerts a protective role against the gram-negative organisms that are important in periodontal diseases.

Three lines of evidence support a central role for the PMNL in the host response. The first line of evidence derives from clinical studies of naturally occurring disease states involving primary and secondary immunodeficiencies. As the predominant phagocyte in blood and inflamed tissues, the PMNL plays a crucial role in the defense process against virulent bacteria. Observations from human and animal studies demonstrate that defective PMNL function is associated with the presence of periodontal destruction (Van Dyke et al, 1987). Although periodontal destruction has been associated with PMNL dysfunction, individuals suffering from primary lymphocyte disorders, such as hereditary deficiencies in cell-mediated immunity, exhibit no greater severity of periodontitis than do healthy persons.

The second line of evidence implicating the PMNL as a major protective cell against oral bacterial pathogens is the observation that several periodontopathic bacteria have significant anti-PMNL virulence factors. *Porphyromonas gingivalis* and *Actinobacillus actinomycetemcomitans* are leukoaggressive; that is, they produce toxins and other factors that either reduce PMNL function or kill PMNLs.

The third line of evidence for the critical role of PMNLs in periodontal diseases comes from the identification of PMNL dysfunction in several forms of early-onset periodontitis, including localized juvenile periodontitis, rapidly progressive periodontitis, and prepubertal periodontitis. There are a large database and extensive literature supporting the role of PMNL abnormalities in localized juvenile periodontitis.

These three lines of evidence lead to the conclusion that normal PMNL function is an important determinant of host resistance to periodontal destruction. Conversely, deficiencies of PMNL function often result in increased susceptibility to periodontitis.

Among chronic diseases, type I diabetes mellitus is considered to be the most important RI, RF, and PRF for periodontal diseases. It is reported that patients with insulin-dependent juvenile diabetes are more susceptible to early onset of local periodontal destruction. This is initially restricted to first molars and incisors but becomes more widespread, affecting other teeth. It seems to be generally agreed that plaque indices in these subjects are similar to those of age-matched nondiabetics and that the severity of the periodontal destruction, when present, is not related to the amount of gingival plaque. A number of defects in host defense systems are described in this disease.

The susceptibility of these diabetic patients to periodontal destruction may be multifactorial and depend on defects of phagocytic cells, such as the PMNL, and on the vascular and structural defects of the periodontal tissues. There are, however, reports of changes in the subgingival flora of these patients, with low numbers of *Porphyromonas gingivalis* and increases in the proportions of *Fusobacterium, Capnocytophaga,* and *Actinomyces naeslundii.* It is unknown whether the altered subgingival flora is due to the diabetic state and might cause the destruction or whether it is secondary to the periodontal destruction.

Even in adults, a close relationship has been shown between diabetes mellitus and periodontal diseases. In a large cross-sectional study of adults by Grossi et al (1994), diabetes mellitus was ranked third, after age and smoking, as a risk indicator for severe forms of periodontal disease. In addition, it was the only systemic disease positively associated with attachment loss. This association was valid even after corrections were made for age, smoking, socioeconomic factors, plaque, and calculus. Diabetics were twice as likely as nondiabetics to exhibit attachment loss (odds ratio 2.3).

CHAPTER 5

RISK PROFILES FOR TOOTH LOSS, DENTAL CARIES, AND PERIODONTAL DISEASES

RISK PROFILES: A TOOL FOR PREDICTING RISK AND COMMUNICATING WITH PATIENTS

Risk profiles for tooth loss, dental caries, and periodontal diseases can be graphically visualized (manually or by computer) by combining symptoms of disease (prevalence, incidence, treatment needs, etc); etiologic factors; external modifying risk indicators, risk factors, and prognostic risk factors; internal modifying risk indicators, risk factors, and prognostic risk factors; and preventive factors. The degree of risk, designated as 0, 1, 2, or 3 (ie, 0 = no risk, 3 = high risk) is indicated by green, blue, yellow, and red, respectively. The graphs should also be used as a tool for communication with the patient when discussing the oral health status, etiology, modifying factors, prevention, possibilities, responsibilities, and reevaluations.

RISK PROFILES FOR TOOTH LOSS

The risk for future tooth loss can be evaluated by combining several risk indicators, risk factors, and prognostic risk factors. Among these are age, estimated risk for periodontal diseases (P0 to P3) and dental caries (C0 to C3), poor socioeconomic conditions, chronic diseases, iatrogenic root fractures, trauma, genetics, impaired host response, medication, and irregular dental care habits.

Figure 32 illustrates evaluation of the risk profile for tooth loss. In many industrialized countries, elderly people have heavily restored dentitions because of high caries incidence 30 to 50 years previously. Their dental treatment comprised "drilling, filling, and billing." In such populations, the most frequent reason for tooth loss would be iatrogenic root fractures because of posts in endodontically treated teeth. On the other hand, in developing countries with very limited oral health care resources, the main reasons for tooth loss would be untreated periodontal diseases and dental caries among elderly people and untreated dental caries and trauma among young people.

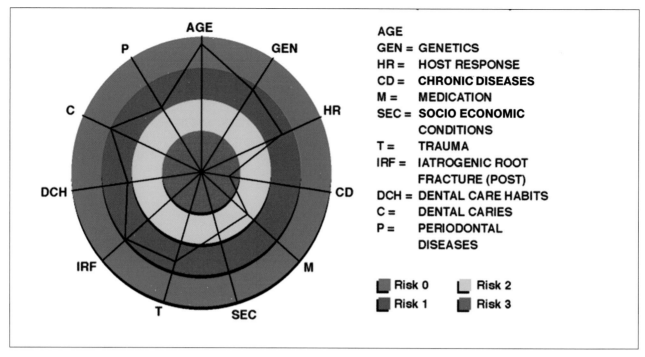

Fig 32 Risk profile for tooth loss (TL0–TL3).

RISK PROFILES FOR DENTAL CARIES AND PERIODONTAL DISEASES

Risk profiles for dental caries and periodontal diseases can be designed in combination or separately. Figure 33 illustrates a combined risk profile from a patient who, after the first detailed examination and history taking, was classified as a high-risk patient for dental caries as well as periodontal diseases (C3P3). This assessment was made on the following basis:

1. His prevalence of caries and periodontitis was high.
2. His incidence of caries and periodontitis used to be very high.
3. He was exposed to many etiologic factors—both nonspecific factors (high plaque formation rate and plaque volume) and specific caries-inducing pathogens and periopathogens (mutans streptococci, *Lactobacillus*, *Actinobacillus*

actinomycetemcomitans, Porphyromonas gingivalis, Bacteroides forsythus, Prevotella intermedia, and *Treponema denticola*).
4. He also exhibited many external and internal modifying risk indicators, risk factors, and prognostic risk factors for both dental caries and periodontal diseases.

After case presentation and self-diagnosis, the sharing of responsibilities by the patient (the owner of the oral cavity) and the oral health personnel was discussed.

Two years later, he was classified as a low-risk patient for both dental caries and periodontal diseases (C1P1), on the following basis:

1. The etiologic factors had been dramatically reduced (from red to green) as a result of an initial intensified combination of mechanical and chemical plaque control (self-care and professional) and maintenance of a high standard of plaque control, ie, a dramatic improvement in the most important preventive factors.

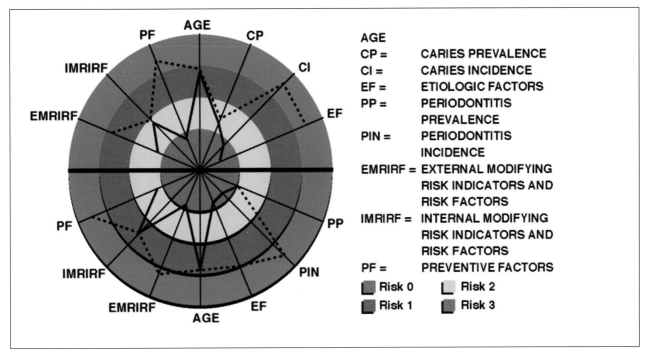

Fig 33 Risk profile for dental caries and periodontal diseases. (solid line) C3P3; (dotted line) C1P1.

2. Initial treatment needs (excavation and restoration of open cavities, scaling, root planing, and debridement of diseased periodontal pockets) were fulfilled, and plaque-retentive factors were eliminated.

3. Important external modifying risk indicators and risk factors were reduced. The patient stopped smoking and reduced the estimated daily sugar clearance time by 80%.

4. The use of fluorides was improved. A new fluoride toothpaste technique was introduced, and use of fluoride chewing gum after meals was recommended. This was supplemented with professional application of fluoride varnish.

As a consequence of the improved preventive measures and healthier lifestyle, the patient developed no new carious lesions (caries incidence changed from red to green) and experienced no further loss of periodontal support (periodontitis incidence changed from red to green) (see Fig 33).

If the patients are predominantly at high risk for only dental caries or periodontal disease, a more detailed risk profile is designed for the specific disease.

CHAPTER 6

PLAQUE CONTROL FOR THE PREVENTION OF ORAL DISEASES

Among preventive factors, plaque control must be ranked number one, because it is directed toward the cause of gingivitis and periodontitis as well as dental caries, namely, the pathogenic microflora that colonize the tooth surfaces and form dental plaque biofilms (in other words, the sole etiologic factors of the aforementioned oral diseases). This also has been confirmed in animal and human studies (Keyes, 1960; Löe et al, 1965; von der Fehr et al, 1970; Lindhe et al, 1973). Germ-free animals frequently fed with sugar do not develop caries until they are infected by cariogenic microflora, which colonize their tooth surfaces. Studies in humans have shown that high-quality plaque control can prevent and control gingivitis, periodontitis, and dental caries in children as well as adults (for review, see Axelsson, 1994, 1998).

Plaque control can be achieved mechanically or chemically by self-care or professionally by dentists or dental hygienists. Plaque control programs based on needs-related combinations of these methods are, to date, the most successful means for prevention of gingivitis, marginal periodontitis, and dental caries. (For review, see Axelsson, 1998.)

MECHANICAL PLAQUE CONTROL

Self-care

The effectiveness of plaque control by self-care depends on motivation, knowledge, oral hygiene instruction, oral hygiene aids, and manual dexterity. A huge assortment of oral hygiene aids are available; the dentist or the dental hygienist should assess the individual needs of the patient and recommend appropriate aids.

Toothbrushing

Toothbrushing is the most widely used mechanical means of personal plaque control in the world. For example, almost 100% of Swedish schoolchildren brush their teeth at least once or twice a day, and no fewer than 99.5% of all dentate adults use a toothbrush (Kuusela et al, 1997; Axelsson and Paulander, 1994).

Enthusiastic use of the toothbrush is not, however, synonymous with a high standard of oral hygiene. The toothbrush has very limited access to the wide approximal surfaces of the molars and premolars. Clinical, visual assessment of plaque removal by toothbrushing does not mean that all bacteria have been removed from the tooth surfaces (Fig 34).

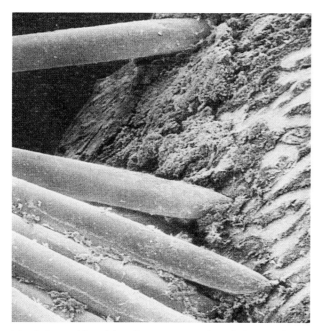

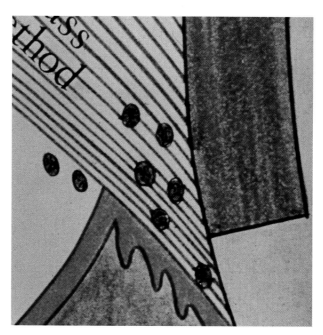

Fig 34 Toothbrush bristles removing dental plaque. (From L. Nilsson. Used with permission.)(Original magnification x 20.)

Fig 35 Bass method of toothbrushing. (From J. Waerhaug. Reprinted with permission of the University of Oslo.)

To systematize the toothbrushing procedure, different methods have been recommended. At least during the last decades, the Bass method has been the most frequently recommended (Bass, 1954). Experimentally, it has been shown that proper use of the Bass method, three times per week, will prevent formation of subgingival plaque on buccal surfaces accessible to the toothbrush and that plaque can be removed at least 1 mm subgingivally (Waerhaug, 1981a) (Fig 35).

However, studies comparing the plaque-removing effect of different toothbrushing methods have shown that, with all methods, the effect on the approximal tooth surfaces is very limited, particularly in the molar and premolar regions (Gjermo and Flötra, 1970). Therefore, the toothbrushing procedure has to be supplemented with special interproximal toothcleaning aids, such as dental floss or tape, toothpicks, and interdental brushes.

Especially for handicapped people and young children, electric toothbrushes are very useful. The rotating pointed interspace brush (Rotadent) is especially useful for cleaning the approximal surfaces in open approximal spaces and for cleaning the fissures of erupting molars (Figs 36 and 37). Another relatively new device (Fig 38) has a round brush head with a 70-degree back-and-forth movement (Oral-B–Braun). It has shown promising results compared to regular manual toothbrushes. Ultrasonically powered toothbrushes are also available, as are devices with a multiset of pointed brushes rotating in different directions (Interplak). (For reviews, see Van der Weijden et al, 1998.)

On the approximal surfaces of molars and premolars, use of a flat, fluoridated dental tape combined with a fluoride toothpaste is recommended for children and young adults. By applying the so-called rubbing-technique, either holding the tape by hand or in a special holder, it is possible to remove plaque 2 mm subgingivally on the approximal surfaces of the molars (Waerhaug, 1981b) (Figs 39 and 40).

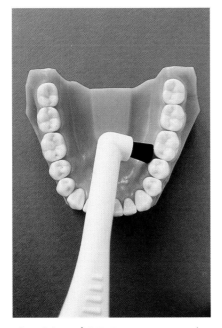
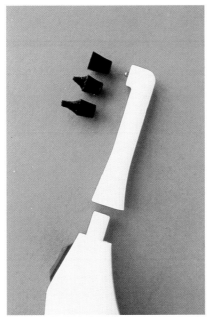
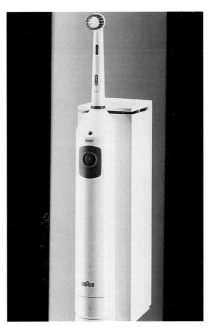

Figs 36 and 37 Rotating pointed interspace toothbrush (Rotadent), useful for cleaning approximal surfaces in open approximal spaces and the fissures of erupting molars.

Fig 38 Electric toothbrush (Oral-B – Braun) with a round brush head and 70-degree back-and-forth movement.

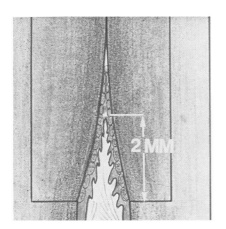
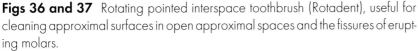
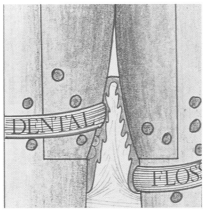

Figs 39 and 40 Plaque removal from the approximal surfaces of molars. Flat, fluoridated dental tape, used in a rubbing technique, can remove 2 mm of subgingival plaque. (From J. Waerhaug. Reprinted with permission of the University of Oslo.)

Figure 41 is a typical bitewing radiograph from a Scandinavian adult, about 50 years old. The patient has approximal restorations with some subgingival overhangs, secondary caries, and some loss of alveolar bone. The location of the gingival margin and papillae are marked, and in situ placement of two pointed (wedge-shaped and triangular) toothpicks in the mandibular teeth is illustrated.

It has been shown in vivo, and at autopsy, that a pointed, triangular toothpick inserted inter-proximally can maintain a plaque-free region 2 to 3 mm subgingivally (Fig 42) (Morch and Waerhaug, 1956). The resilience of the gingival papilla allows cleaning apical to the subgingival margins of restorations (ie, risk surfaces for recurrent caries). For prevention and control of periodontitis and approximal secondary caries in molars and premolars, this subgingival removal of approximal plaque is probably more important than the supragingival cleaning. Therefore, a fluoridated, pointed, triangular toothpick is the most

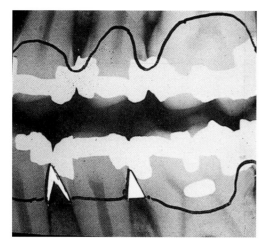 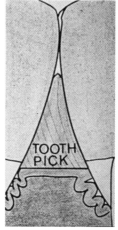

Fig 41 (left) Bitewing radiograph of a 50-year-old Scandinavian. The location of the gingival margin and papillae is marked. Placement of two pointed (wedge-shaped and triangular) toothpicks is illustrated.

Fig 42 (right) Triangular pointed toothpick inserted interdentally. Because of the resilience of the papillae, plaque biofilms can be removed 2 to 3 mm subgingivally. Delivery of fluoride from toothpaste is also enhanced by depression of the gingival papilla.

Fig 43 Tailor-made interdental brush as it should look.

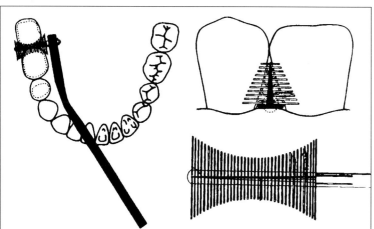

suitable oral hygiene aid for approximal tooth-cleaning in adults.

The best time to apply the cleaning power of toothpaste as a fluoride vehicle is just as the gingival papilla is depressed (Figs 41 and 42). In individuals with advanced periodontal disease, with wide interdental spaces and partially exposed root surfaces, interdental brushes are recommended. Most interdental brushes are circular in cross section. The effect would probably be enhanced if the brush were triangular instead of circular (Fig 43) (Axelsson, 1981). Other special supplementary oral hygiene aids are interspace toothbrushes for tipped or rotated teeth, Superfloss (Oral-B) for cleaning around fixed partial denture pontics, and tongue scrapers.

Establishment of needs-related oral hygiene habits

A fundamental principle of all preventive action is that the positive effect is greatest where the risk for disease is greatest. The patient has the greatest chance of being able to see positive results in his or her oral hygiene efforts if he or she concentrates initially on key-risk teeth and key-risk surfaces—ie, in a toothbrushing population—the approximal surfaces of the molars and premolars. However, interdental cleaning is practically nonexistent and not an established habit in most countries. Based on studies of normal plaque distribution, the rate and pattern of plaque re-formation on cleaned teeth, and dental disease in the dentition and on individual tooth surfaces, it may be stated that, in toothbrushing populations, needs-related toothcleaning is currently not practiced. The adult patient today tends to clean principally those tooth surfaces least susceptible to disease. In other words, there is a large unexploited source of dental care that must be tapped. Yet of 8,760 hours per year, the individual patient normally spends no more than 2 hours in the dental clinic.

The first condition for success in attempting to establish needs-related toothcleaning habits is a well-motivated, well-informed, and well-instructed patient. *Motivation* is defined as readiness to act or the driving force behind a person's actions. Greater responsibility has been described as the motivating factor of longest duration. People's actions are also governed by the needs that they feel they have. Therefore, training of the patient in self-diagnosis is of greatest importance.

In this context, risk profiles and a toothcleaning chart (Fig 44) are useful tools. On the basis of the joint (patient-professional) observations of disease factors outlined on the risk profile and the toothcleaning chart, the Plaque Formation Rate Index (PFRI), and the location of plaque in the patient's mouth, the patient should be encouraged to make suggestions as to the choice of oral hygiene aids and, above all, the order of priorities for cleaning.

Thereafter, it is extremely important that the division of responsibility be discussed. The primary responsibility of the patient (the owner of the oral cavity) is the daily care of the teeth. The necessary methods should be specified. When the division of responsibility is complete, a "contract" could be drawn up and signed by the parties involved. The responsibility ensuing from an agreement that an individual has put his or her name to is more binding than a hasty affirmative given in a moment of suddenly inspired courage.

As already mentioned, a fundamental prerequisite for establishing needs-related toothcleaning habits is a well-motivated, well-informed, and well-instructed patient. However, studies in behavioral science show that there is still a high risk that these habits will not become firmly estab-

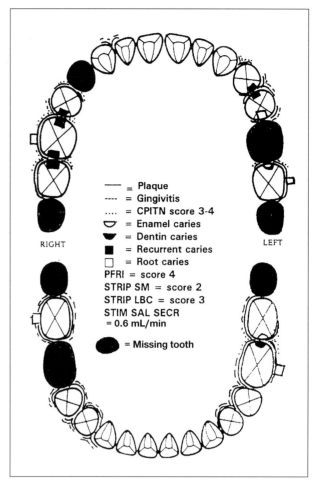

Fig 44 Sample toothcleaning chart. (CPITN) Community Periodontal Index of Treatment Needs; (PFRI) Plaque Formation Rate Index; (SM) *Streptococcus mutans*; (LBC) *Lactobacillus* count; (STIM SAL SECR) stimulated salivary flow rate.

lished. Therefore, when new habits are established, they should be linked very firmly to already established habits. The new habit should always be carried out immediately prior to the established habit, because the risk that the latter will not be performed is minimal.

These principles of behavioral science are called the *linking method* and have been described in a dental context (Weinstein and Getz, 1978). If the patient has irregular oral hygiene habits, an interview should reveal already-established habits that, in terms of frequency and point in time during the day, happen to coincide well with the proposed oral hygiene routine. According to the linking method, oral hygiene should be "slotted in" to the patient's daily routine but immediately prior to it. For example, needs-related toothcleaning in patients with well-established daily toothbrushing habits should start with interproximal cleaning in the molar and premolar regions, before they use the toothbrush.

These principles for establishment of needs-related oral hygiene habits were implemented recently in a 3-year longitudinal study. Twelve-year-old schoolchildren in São Paulo, Brazil, were randomly assigned to one of two test groups or one control group. All the children had a well-established habit of daily toothbrushing with a fluoride toothpaste and were exposed to fluoridated drinking water (Axelsson et al, 1994).

Children in test group I were trained and activated to identify sites with inflamed gingivae that could heal and sites with enamel caries that could remineralize. Using the PFRI as a guideline, they deduced how frequently they needed to clean their teeth and which sites required special attention during toothcleaning procedures. In accordance with the linking method, they were motivated to apply fluoride toothpaste to the approximal surfaces of molars and premolars first. After these surfaces had been meticulously cleaned with dental tape and a rubbing technique, the patients then carefully cleaned the lingual and buccal surfaces with a toothbrush and fluoride toothpaste. After three initial visits at short intervals, the children were recalled every 3 months for reevaluation of the results based on self-diagnosis.

The children in test group II were trained, both on models and in their mouths, to clean every tooth surface meticulously with dental tape, fluoride toothpaste, and a toothbrush. They were recalled for reinstruction at the same intervals as test group I.

During the 3-year period, the children in test group I developed 60% and 75% fewer new approximal carious lesions in dentin per individual on the molars and premolars, respectively, compared to subjects in test group II and the control group. The conclusions from the study were (1) in a toothbrushing population using fluoride toothpaste and fluoridated drinking water, a highly significant reduction in the incidence of approximal caries will be achieved by an oral hygiene training program based on self-diagnosis and the linking method; and (2) in such a population, frequent repetition of meticulous oral hygiene training is almost redundant (Axelsson et al, 1994). The cost effectiveness of large-scale implementation of the experiences from this low-cost, low-technology study based on self-care would be enormous.

Oral hygiene training based on self-diagnosis and the linking method was also implemented in a 15-year longitudinal study in adults. The strategy was so effective that the intervals between PMTC treatments could successively be extended, while an optimal to suboptimal effect on gingivitis, periodontitis, and dental caries was recorded (Axelsson et al, 1991).

Finally, most dental professionals have observed that high-quality mechanical plaque control by self-care prevents not only gingivitis and periodontitis but also dental caries. Up to the age of 20 years, both my wife and I developed almost the same number of decayed or filled surfaces as the average for the Swedish population. However, since I started dental school in 1955, I have not developed one carious lesion (for almost 45 years), and I have required no scaling because it is not necessary. My wife has developed only one carious lesion during the same period, although before 1970 we had no efficient fluoride toothpaste. Our two grown children, Eva, 38 years old (Fig 45a), and Torbjörn, 35 years old (Fig 45b), are both still caries- and gingivitis-free, although they have our genes, have used no fluoride agents other than a toothpaste, and are without any professional preventive measures, such as fissure sealants, showing that "clean teeth never decay."

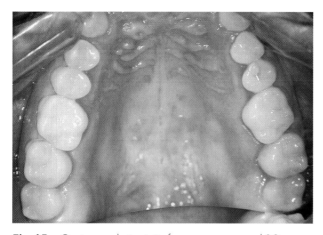

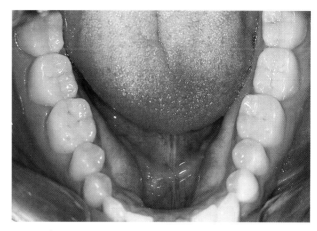

Fig 45a Caries- and gingivitis-free woman, aged 38 years. Meticulous toothcleaning has prevented oral disease, even in the absence of preventive measures such as fissure sealants.

Fig 45b Caries- and gingivitis-free man, aged 35 years.

Professional mechanical toothcleaning (PMTC)

Technique

Professional mechanical toothcleaning, by specially trained personnel (eg, a prophylaxis dental nurse, dental hygienist, or dentist), is the selective removal of plaque—not only supragingivally but also 1 to 3 mm subgingivally—from all tooth surfaces, using mechanically driven instruments and fluoride prophylaxis paste. Therefore, the correct term should be *gingival plaque removal (control)*. If calculus and deep subgingival plaque biofilms are also removed, the procedure is usually referred to as *scaling* or *debridement* and is performed only by dentists and dental hygienists. It must be emphasized that so-called prophylaxis or polishing with a rotating rubber cup and prophylaxis paste, mainly on the buccal, lingual, and occlusal surfaces, ie, the nonrisk surfaces, in a toothbrushing population should not be confused with *professional* mechanical toothcleaning.

In the so-called Karlstad studies in adults and children (Axelsson et al, 1991, 1993a; for review, see Axelsson, 1981, 1994) PMTC was carried out

using the following techniques, which may be regarded as the standard procedure. For PMTC, the following materials are necessary:

1. Plaque-disclosing pellets
2. A Profin contra-angle handpiece (a new, modified EVA prophylaxis contra-angle handpiece; Dentatus) and reciprocating tips
3. A prophylaxis contra-angle handpiece and rotating rubber cup
4. A fluoride-containing prophylaxis paste (medium abrasive)
5. A syringe for injecting the prophylaxis paste interproximally (Fig 46)

Because PMTC must be directed to the tooth surfaces normally neglected by the patient, disclosure of plaque is the first step. Plaque deposits are often heaviest in the mandibular lingual embrasures of the molars and premolars (Fig 47). Plaque is almost always present in the interproximal spaces if continuous visible plaque is found in the line angles. This can be verified by probing.

A disposable syringe facilitates the application of fluoride polishing paste in the interproximal spaces. Approximal application should always be started from the lingual aspect of the mandibular

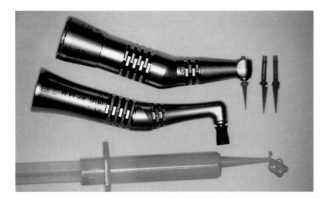

Fig 46 Equipment for professional mechanical tooth-cleaning: (top to bottom) Profin contra-angle handpiece and reciprocating tips; prophylaxis contra-angle handpiece and rotating rubber cup; and a syringe for injecting prophylaxis paste interproximally.

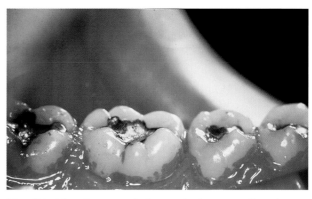

Fig 47 After the use of plaque-disclosing pellets, heavy gingival plaque in the mandibular lingual embrasures of the molars and premolars is visible.

teeth. This is a rational means of applying the fluoride prophylaxis paste to all approximal surfaces. With paste already applied to the surfaces requiring maximum attention, mechanical cleaning can be carried out very quickly (Fig 48a).

The specially designed prophylaxis contra-angle handpiece with reciprocating V-shaped flexible tips or triangular pointed tips is used for interproximal PMTC. The tips are self-steering and reciprocating with 1.0- to 1.5-mm strokes. When entering the interproximal space, the tip will have a 10-degree coronal angle until the papilla is pressed down. Thanks to the resilience of the papillae, a cleaning effect can be expected 2 to 3 mm subgingivally (see Figs 41 and 42).

A suitable speed for the contra-angle handpiece is approximately 7,000 rpm (ie, 14,000 strokes per minute or 250 strokes per second). The direction of the tip should continually be adjusted vertically and horizontally so as to reach the entire approximal surface. At the same time, fluoride polishing paste is applied to all cleaned surfaces.

The PMTC should always commence from the lingual surface of the mandibular molars, according to the linking method (Fig 48b). When the approximal surfaces have been carefully cleaned from the more easily accessible lingual side, they are then cleaned from the buccal direction. The maxillary interproximal surfaces are cleaned next

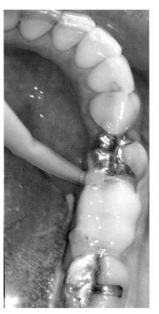
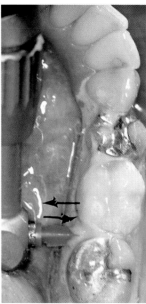

Figs 48a and 48b Professional mechanical toothcleaning after syringed application of fluoride polishing paste. The cleaning always commences from the lingual surfaces of the mandibular molars.

in the same order: lingual embrasures, followed by the buccal. A regular prophylaxis contra-angle handpiece and rotating rubber cup (see Fig 46), combined with the application of the same prophylaxis paste, are recommended for PMTC on the lingual and buccal surfaces.

Hand instruments, such as curettes, may also supplement the aforementioned instruments to remove partly mineralized plaque biofilms in the gingival sulcus as well as more deeply located subgingival plaque biofilms. This method of PMTC is sometimes called *debridement*.

Effectiveness

Although the preventive effect of plaque control programs on gingivitis and periodontitis is generally accepted, the preventive effect of mechanical plaque control on the development of caries has been questioned. We therefore initiated a series of longitudinal plaque control programs, including PMTC, to test the effect of mechanical plaque control on gingivitis and dental caries in schoolchildren.

The first longitudinal clinical trial was initiated to test the hypothesis that gingivitis and dental caries do not develop in schoolchildren maintained on an oral hygiene program that includes PMTC and oral hygiene instruction. During a 4-year period, the test group received PMTC from a preventive dentistry assistant, 16 times a year for the first 2 years and then four to six times a year for the following 2 years. The control group received ordinary dental treatment, including supervised toothbrushing using the Bass method, once a year and fluoride rinsing 10 times a year, for the entire trial period. There were no true negative controls; for ethical reasons, the subjects in the control group were maintained on the regular dental care schedule.

During the 4-year period, the control group developed 15 times more new carious surfaces than the test group. As a consequence of extremely low plaque scores in the test group, the gingival conditions also were excellent (Axelsson and Lindhe, 1977).

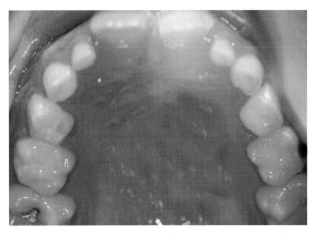

Fig 49a Patient in preventive dentistry test group at baseline, aged 7 years. The patient had one restored maxillary molar.

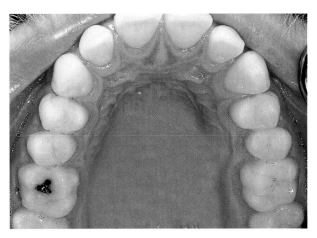

Fig 49b Same patient, aged 18 years. No additional teeth have developed caries.

The long-term effect of early introduction of such a high-quality mechanical plaque control program must not be underestimated. Figures 49 and 50 show two representative patients from the youngest test group, aged 7 years, at baseline. At baseline, the first patient had one restored maxillary molar (Fig 49a). At age 18 years, this patient exhibited no increase in the number of carious or restored teeth (Fig 49b).

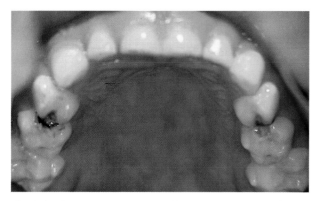

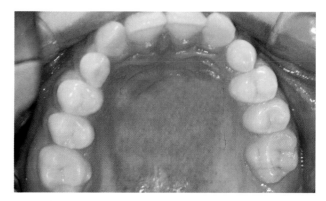

Fig 50a Patient in preventive dentistry test group at baseline, aged 7 years. Several primary teeth are carious.

Fig 50b Same patient, aged 12 years. All permanent teeth are caries free.

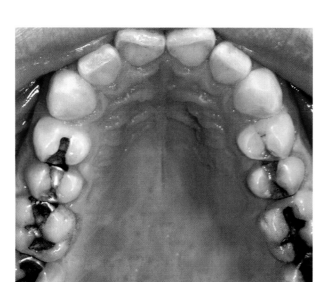

Fig 51 Typical patient in control group, aged 18 years. All the permanent premolars and molars have restorations.

Figure 50a shows the second patient at baseline with numerous carious primary teeth. One year after the end of the study, all the permanent teeth were caries free (Fig 50b). In contrast, Fig 51 shows a representative patient from the control group, 7 years after the end of the study, at the age of 18 years, with most approximal surfaces of the posterior teeth restored.

This study was followed by numerous clinical trials to compare the separate effect of PMTC on caries and gingivitis to the effect of other preventive measures, such as oral hygiene training, chemical plaque control, and topical use of fluorides. In all these studies, frequent PMTC was superior to the other measures (Axelsson et al, 1976; Axelsson and Lindhe, 1981). The first Karlstad study

based on PMTC aroused interest in other countries, such as Norway, Denmark, Great Britain, and Brazil. They too followed up and carried out PMTC-based studies, mostly with similar results (for review, see Axelsson, 1981; Bellini et al, 1981; Gjermo, 1986; Axelsson, 1994). For cost effectiveness, however, it is important that the frequency of PMTC be based on individual needs.

Frequent PMTC has also been successfully used in maintenance programs after initial nonsurgical or surgical treatment of marginal periodontitis. In a study by Rosling et al (1976), patients with a high prevalence of infrabony pockets were randomly allotted to a test or a control group. After initial open flap surgery, scaling, and root planing, the test group received PMTC every second week during a 2-year period. At reexamination, about 95% of the infrabony pockets had healed and the gingival condition was excellent.

So-called supragingival plaque control is considered to have little effect on the subgingival microflora of deep periodontal pockets. However, this may not be true for PMTC in moderately deep pockets (4 to 6 mm). A series of studies has shown that the pocket depth and the total number of subgingival microflora gradually decreased in such pockets as a result of frequent PMTC without prior subgingival scaling. In addition, there was a shift from a periopathogenic to a less pathogenic microflora (for reviews, see Axelsson, 1994; Kieser, 1994). These facts may be explained as an effect of the repeated 2- to 3-mm subgingival plaque removal accomplished (see Figs 40 to 42) by PMTC, in contrast to supragingival plaque control.

The most cost-effective course for treatment and control of periodontal diseases would be an initial, comprehensive, subgingival, "nonaggressive" scaling, root planing, and debridement, followed by a maintenance program based on excellent control of gingival plaque by a combination of self-care and PMTC at needs-related intervals.

These principles were tested in a 15-year longitudinal study in adults (Axelsson et al, 1991). Two groups of subjects from one geographic area were recruited. Three hundred seventy-five were assigned to a test group and 180 to a control group, stratified into three age groups: 20 to 35 years, 36 to 50 years, and 51 to 70 years. During the first 6-year period, the control patients were seen regularly once a year and given traditional dental care. After initial nonaggressive scaling, root planing, and debridement, the test group participants were seen every other month for the first 2 years, and once every third month for the following 4 years. They were educated individually in proper oral hygiene technique, based on self-diagnosis, and received PMTC, supplemented by debridement, where necessary, by a dental hygienist.

Reexaminations were carried out toward the end of the third and sixth years of the study. On average, the control group lost 1.2 mm of peri-odontal attachment per individual, while the test group lost none at all. Although most of the subjects in the control group did not lose any periodontal attachment, the condition of some subjects deteriorated badly, with continued attachment loss and development of new carious surfaces (Axelsson and Lindhe, 1978, 1981). For ethical reasons, after the 6-year period, the control group was also offered need-related preventive dentistry, and many accepted.

All test subjects then received an individualized secondary preventive program by the same dental hygienist for the following 9-year period, up to the 15-year reexamination. To maximize cost effectiveness, the intervals, as well as the preventive measures used, were based strictly on individual needs. Approximately 65% visited the dental hygienist only once a year, 30% twice a year, and 5% (the high-risk individuals) three to six times a year.

Only 0.23 teeth were lost per individual over 15 years. These results could be extrapolated to imply that a 50-year-old subject offered such a program would be more than 100 years old before losing another single tooth. During the same period of time (15 years), it is estimated that the Swedish adult population lost, on average, two to three teeth per individual.

During the entire 15-year period, there was a mean gain of 0.3 mm of probing periodontal attachment per individual and less than one new carious surface developed per individual, regardless of age. Caries incidence and periodontal attachment gain were about the same in the 66 to 85 year olds as in the 36 to 50 year olds. In addition, it was estimated that the annual costs for dental care in the test group were only about 50% of the average annual costs for Swedish adult patients (Axelsson et al, 1991).

The long-term effect on tooth loss, caries prevalence, loss of periodontal support, gingival health status, and standard of oral hygiene may be illustrated by three patients—one from each age group—exhibiting more loss of periodontal support than the average for the age group at the baseline examination in 1972.

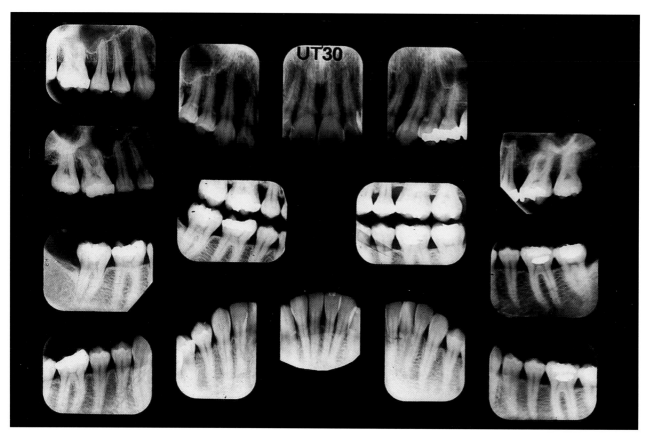

Fig 52 Complete-mouth radiographs of a 30-year-old woman in test group 1 (professional mechanical toothcleaning) at the baseline examination (1972). Early-onset periodontitis has resulted in loss of periodontal support around the maxillary first molars.

Figures 52 and 53 show complete-mouth radiographs of a woman from test group 1 at the age of 30, in 1972, and at the age of 45, in 1987. As an effect of early-onset localized periodontitis, in 1972 the patient had greater-than-average loss of periodontal support for her age, around the maxillary first molars. During the following 15 years no teeth were lost, there was no further loss of periodontal support, and no new carious lesions developed.

Figures 54 and 55 show the buccogingival health status and level of oral hygiene at the 15-year reexamination. For esthetic reasons, many of the 25 to 30 amalgam restorations could have been replaced, for example with ceramic crowns, onlays, or inlays, but the patient chose to invest in preventive rather than restorative dentistry.

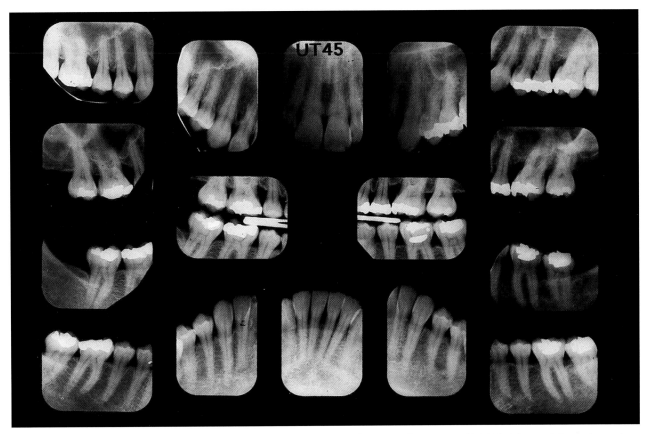

Fig 53 Complete-mouth radiographs of the patient in Fig 52, at the age of 45 years (1987). No teeth have been lost, there has been no further loss of periodontal support, and no new carious lesions have developed.

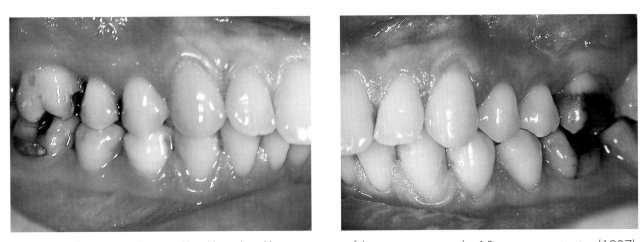

Figs 54 and 55 Buccal gingival health and oral hygiene status of the same patient at the 15-year reexamination (1987).

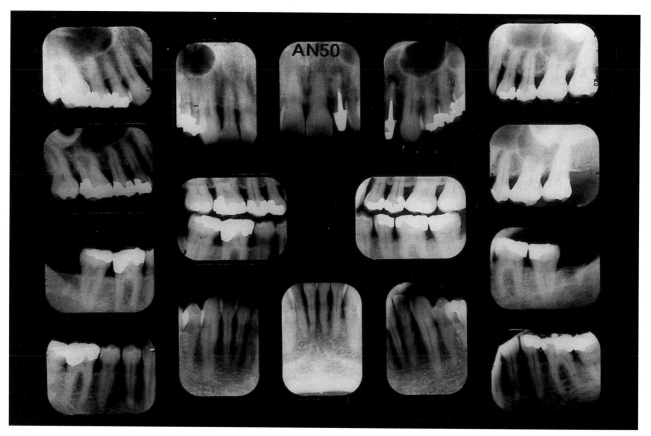

Fig 56 Complete-mouth radiographs of a 50-year-old man in test group 2 (professional mechanical toothcleaning) at the baseline examination (1972). He has greater-than-average loss of periodontal support for his age, especially in the maxillary teeth.

Complete-mouth radiographs of a man in test group 2, aged 50 at the baseline examination in 1972, are shown in Fig 56. Radiographs taken at the 15-year reexamination are shown in 1987 (Fig 57). In 1972, the patient exhibited greater-than-average probing attachment loss for his age, especially in the maxillary teeth. During the following 15 years, no teeth were lost, there was no further loss of probing attachment, and no new carious lesions developed.

The buccal gingival health status and level of oral hygiene at the 15-year reexamination are shown in Figs 58 and 59.

Complete-mouth radiographs of a 56-year-old woman in test group 3 at the baseline examination are shown in Fig 60a. The same patient, aged 71, is shown in Fig 60b, taken at the 15-year reexamination. Without a doubt, the number of remaining teeth and the level of remaining periodontal support in 1972 were far below the average for 56 year olds. During the following 15 years, no teeth were lost, no further loss of periodontal attachment was recorded, and no carious lesions were detected.

The patient's oral health status at the age of 77 years is illustrated in complete-mouth radiographs from 1993 (Fig 61). Close-up radiographs of the maxillary right second premolar (tooth 15) in 1972 and 1993 are shown in Figs 62 and 63, respectively. The buccal gingival health status and the level of oral hygiene are shown in Figs 64 and 65, taken 20 years after the baseline examination, at the age of 76 years.

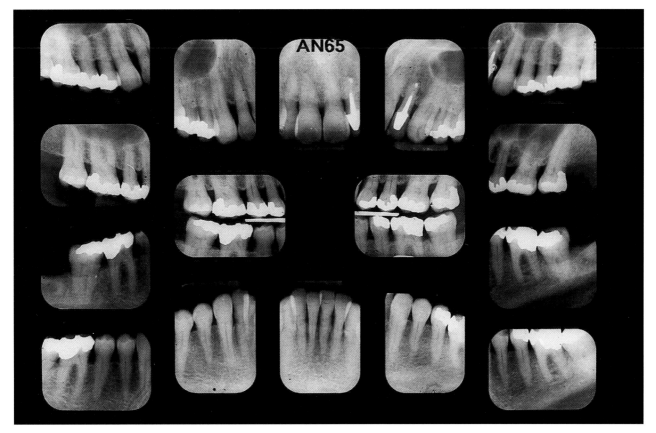

Fig 57 Complete-mouth radiographs of the patient in Fig 56, aged 65 years, at the 15-year reexamination (1987). No teeth have been lost, there has been no further loss of probing attachment level, and no new carious lesions have developed. Observe the well-mineralized margin of the alveolar bone, indicating an absence of active periodontitis.

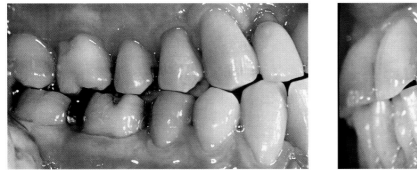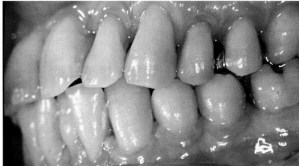

Figs 58 and 59 Buccogingival health and oral hygiene status of the same patient at the 15-year reexamination (1987).

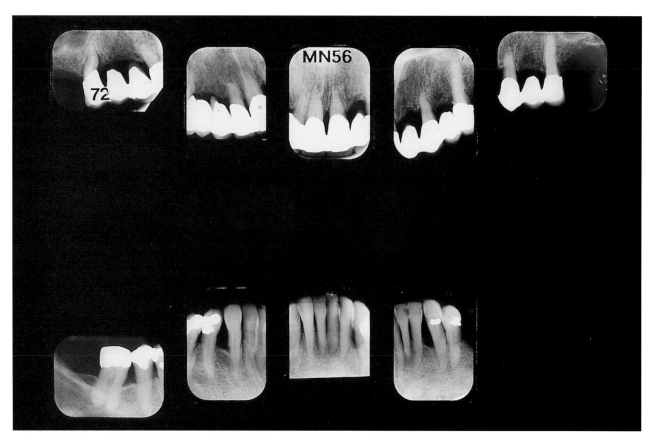

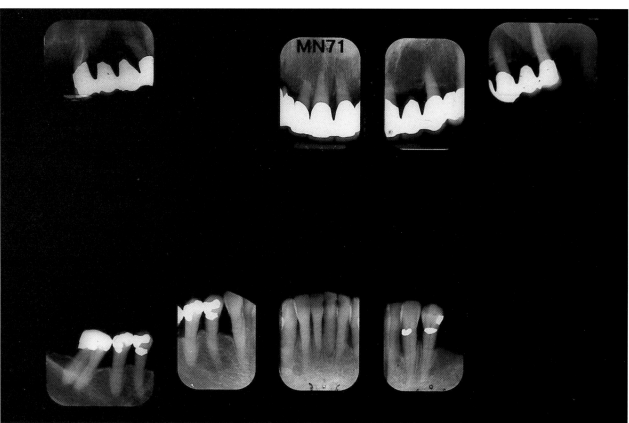

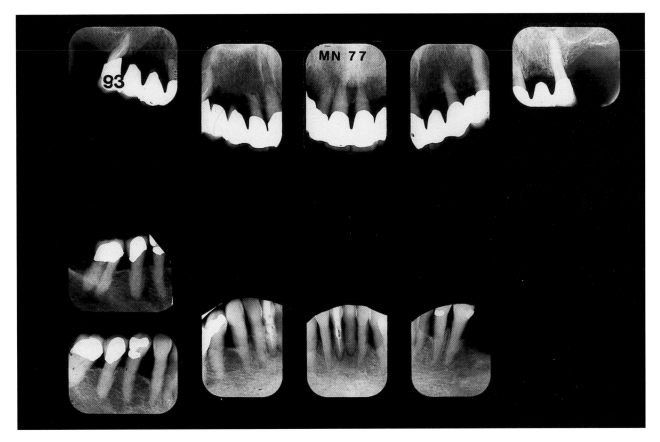

Fig 60a (top left) Complete-mouth radiographs of a 56-year-old woman in test group 3 (professional mechanical toothcleaning) at the baseline examination (1972). The number of remaining teeth and the amount of remaining periodontal support are much less than average for her age group.

Fig 60b (bottom left) Complete-mouth radiographs of the patient in Fig 60a, aged 71 years, at the 15-year reexamination (1987). No additional teeth have been lost, no further loss of probing attachment level has been recorded, and no carious lesions have been detected. Compare the bone level on the mesial surface of the maxillary right second premolar (tooth 15) and the distal surface of the mandibular right canine (tooth 43) to that exhibited in 1972 (Fig 60a).

Fig 61 (above) Complete-mouth radiographs of the same patient, aged 77 years (1993).

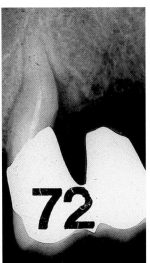

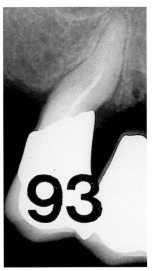

Fig 62 Radiograph of the maxillary right second premolar in 1972.

Fig 63 Radiograph of the maxillary right second premolar in 1993.

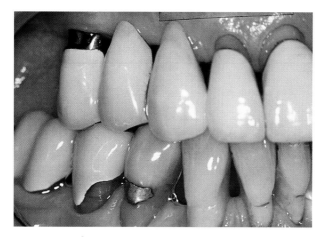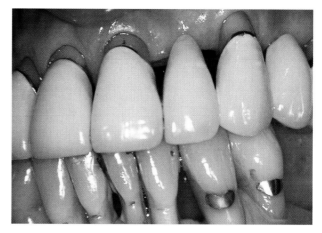

Figs 64 and 65 Buccal gingival health and oral hygiene status of the same patient, aged 76 years, at the 20-year re-examination. The maxillary fixed prosthesis, more than 20 years old, is still intact, without recurrent caries.

Plaque-retentive factors

For optimal mechanical plaque control, through self-care or PMTC, plaque-retentive factors must be eliminated or at least minimized. Plaque-retentive factors occur subgingivally as well as supragingivally. The following conditions, pre-disposing to subgingival plaque retention, may complicate subgingival plaque control:

1. Deep, narrow bony pockets
2. Furcation involvement
3. Root grooves
4. Rough, unplaned cementum
5. Cementum hypoplasia
6. Root resorption
7. Calculus
8. Iatrogenic effects of subgingival scaling, such as grooves and exposed dentinal tubules on the root surfaces
9. Restoration overhangs, defective and ill-fitting crown margins, excess resin cement, and un-polished restorations
10. Recurrent caries and root caries

Supragingival plaque retention is most commonly the result of the following conditions:

1. Caries
2. Restoration overhangs and defective margins
3. Ill-fitting crown and inlay margins
4. Excess resin cement
5. Unpolished restorations
6. Resin composite restorations
7. Supragingival calculus
8. Exposed, unplaned root surfaces

Overhangs are usually located on the approximal surfaces, and mostly subgingivally. Several studies have shown a close relationship between the size of the overhang and local loss of periodontal support as a result of plaque retention (for reviews, see Axelsson, 1994; Kieser, 1994). This is exemplified in Fig 66.

To prevent and control secondary caries and periodontitis through mechanical gingival plaque control, it is much more important that subgingival approximal restorations be optimally finished and repeatedly polished than occlusal, buccal, and lingual restorations. Rotating instruments have traditionally been used to finish and polish restorations and remove overhangs. However, in narrow, triangular interproximal spaces, the subgingival area is almost inaccessible to rotating instruments. Many subgingival approximal restora-

Fig 66 Overhanging restoration (arrow), related to the localized loss of periodontal support.

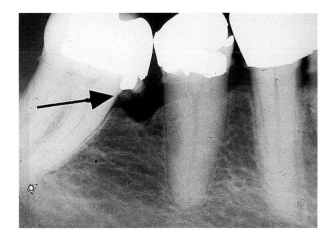

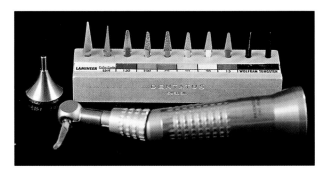

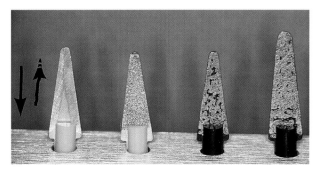

Figs 67 and 68 Reciprocating, thin, spatulate or pointed double–knife-edged instruments, useful for finishing and recontouring restorations and removing overhangs (Profin contra-angle and tips).

tions are therefore poorly finished and have persistent overhangs. As illustrated in Figs 41 and 42, reciprocating triangular or V-shaped pointed instruments are more appropriate for narrow triangular interproximal spaces than are rotating instruments. Because of the resilience of the papillae, such reciprocating instruments can access 2 to 3 mm subgingivally.

Reciprocating, thin, spatulate or pointed double–knife-edged instruments (Figs 67 and 68) are even more useful for finishing, removing overhangs, and recontouring, because they can be used subgingivally between the papillae and the tooth surface. Both diamond-coated and tungsten-coated tips are available in sizes from 15 to 150 μm. Tungsten-coated tips do not harm the tooth enamel, root surfaces, or porcelain or glass-ceramic restorations and are therefore suitable for

final finishing of restorations and removal of excess resin cement.

Figure 69 shows approximal amalgam overhangs that were easily removed (Fig 70) by using the Profin contra-angle and a 50-μm diamond-coated reciprocating tip. Thereafter, the approximal surfaces were finished and polished using less abrasive tips, V-shaped pointed plastic tips, and fluoride prophylaxis paste, successively. Figure 71 illustrates the difference between the use of rotating instruments and thin, double–knife-edged instruments for removal of subgingival approximal excess cement. In contrast to rotating instruments, the reciprocating tips can also be used with a rubber dam in place (Fig 72).

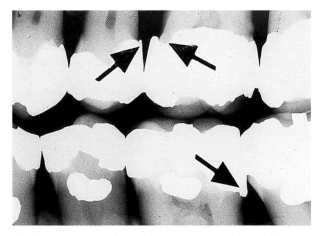

Fig 69 Approximal amalgam overhangs (arrows).

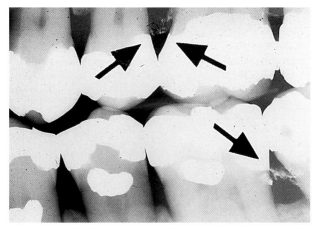

Fig 70 Smoothed margins (arrows), after removal of overhangs with the Profin contra-angle handpiece and a 50-mm diamond-coated reciprocating tip (1.0- to 1.5-mm strokes).

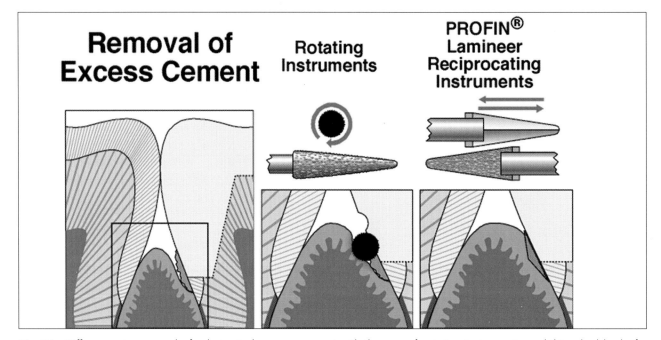

Fig 71 Difference in removal of subgingival excess cement with the use of rotating instruments and thin, double–knife-edged instruments.

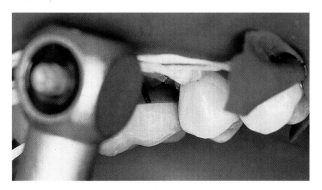

Fig 72 Use of reciprocating tips in the presence of a rubber dam.

Figs 73a and 73b Extremely excessive calculus formation covers the entire distal root of an extracted, untreatable mandibular first molar.

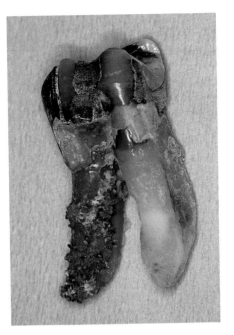

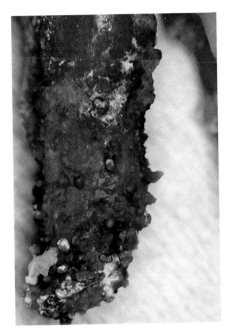

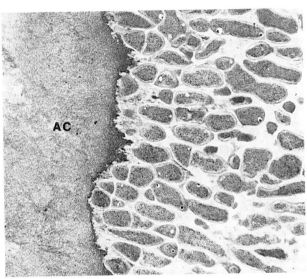

Fig 74 Cross section demonstrating attachment of microflora to the rough outer surface of the root cementum. (From M. Listgarten, 1976. Reprinted with permission.)

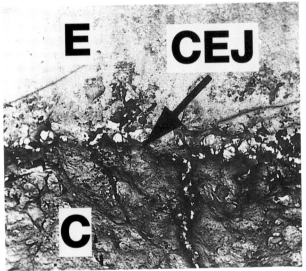

Fig 75 Section demonstrating that the root cementum (C) is much rougher than the enamel (E). The cementoenamel junction (CEJ) also has great plaque-retentive potential.

To inhibit plaque retention, calculus (Figs 73a and 73b) has to be removed by scaling, and the rough outer surface of the root cementum has to planed. Figure 74 illustrates how well the subgingival microflora attaches to the rough outer surface of the root cementum. The root cementum is much rougher than the enamel (Fig 75). The cementoenamel junction (CEJ) is also an anatomic feature with great plaque-retentive potential.

Clinically, the dilemma is that the thickness of the root cementum is only 30 to 100 µm (0.03 to 0.10 mm) on the coronal part of the root. Studies have shown that only 10 to 20 strokes with a sharp hand curette (Coldiron et al, 1990) and a few seconds' application of extra fine-grit (15 µm) rotating diamond scaling tips (Ritz et al, 1992) may result in complete removal of the root cementum, exposing the root dentin and the dentinal tubules.

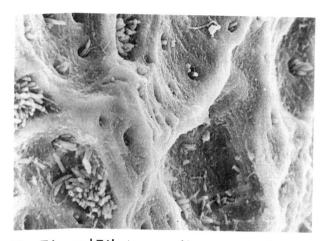
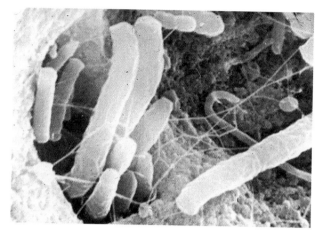

Figs 76a and 76b Invasion of bacteria in the dentinal tubules. (Original magnification x 800 for Fig 76a and x 8000 for Fig 76b.) (From P. A. Adriaens. Reprinted with permission.)

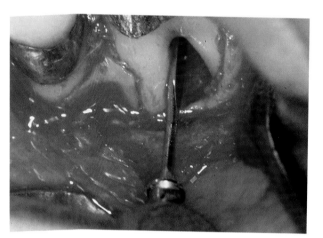

Fig 77

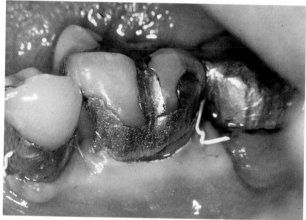

Fig 78

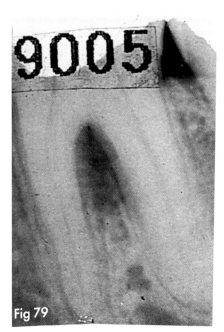

Fig 79

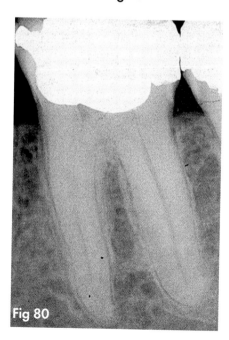

Fig 80

Figs 77 to 80 Use of a non-resorbable barrier membrane (Gore-Tex) in a mandibular molar with degree II to degree III furcation involvement. (From Heden and Axelsson. A case report [unpublished data].)

This allows bacteria to invade the dentinal tubules (Figs 76a and 76b) and even to reach the pulp (Adriaens et al, 1988a, 1988b). Infected root canals may impair the healing of periodontal pockets if the root dentin is not covered by root cementum (Ehnevid et al, 1993a, 1995).

Retaining the root cementum and ensuring its cleanliness are also important for successful regeneration of periodontal support. Examples of successful regeneration are shown in Figs 77 to 86. Figures 77 to 80 show the use of nonresorbable barriers (Gore-Tex, WL Gore) in a mandibular molar with degree II to degree III furcation involvement. Figures 81 to 86 show the use of matrix-guided material (Emdogain gel, Biora) on one- and two-wall bony defects.

For effective elimination of subgingival plaque-retentive factors and the microflora by scaling, root planing, and debridement, and to minimize iatrogenic defects, a sharp universal curette should be used as a probe for identification of calculus; whenever located, calculus should be carefully "lifted away" as a first step. A piezoelectric sonic scaler can also be used for a gross scaling. However, for the final scaling, root planing, and debridement, the choice of instrument should be as nonaggressive as possible.

Figure 87 illustrates the difference between aggressive and nonaggressive instruments for scaling, root planing and debridement. The reciprocating PER-IO-TOR instruments with plane, load-relieving surfaces between essentially right-angled cutting edges are examples of nonaggressive instruments (Fig 88). Because of the special design, once the root cementum is planed, and thereby clean, no further root cementum will be removed. Different shapes and sizes facilitate access on concave and convex surfaces as well as in furcation areas. The reciprocating instruments are used in the Profin contra-angle handpiece (Fig 88). Rotating instruments that work based on the same principles are also available (Figs 89 and 90).

Summary

1. Needs-related oral hygiene habits can be established by self-diagnosis, the linking method, education, and training.
2. High-quality mechanical plaque control through self-care and frequent PMTC will remove plaque biofilms not only supragingivally but also 1 to 3 mm subgingivally, and successfully prevent regrowth of subgingival plaque biofilms, ie, provide gingival plaque control.
3. Even in diseased, untreated periodontal pockets, frequent PMTC results in a reduction in the amount of subgingival microflora and a shift in composition to fewer pathogenic microorganisms.
4. Meticulous PMTC should not be confused with so-called prophylaxis and polishing.
5. To allow optimal mechanical plaque control, plaque-retentive factors must be minimized or eliminated.
6. High-quality mechanical plaque control, based on individual needs, can efficiently prevent initiation (primary prevention) as well as recurrence (secondary prevention) of gingivitis, periodontitis, and dental caries, because the method is directed toward the cause of these diseases.

It must be stressed, however, that the range of reported effects in different clinical studies is strongly correlated to the materials and methods used, sample size, and the incidence of the disease in the population. If needs-related, self-care mechanical plaque control habits are established and supplemented by PMTC at needs-related intervals, very significant preventive effects will be achieved in high-risk individuals, compared with a matched, truly negative control group.

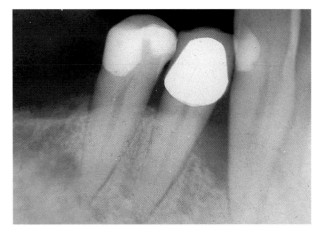

Fig 81

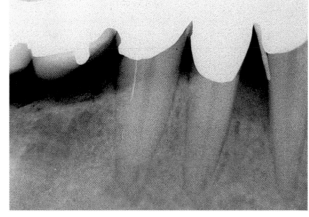

Fig 82

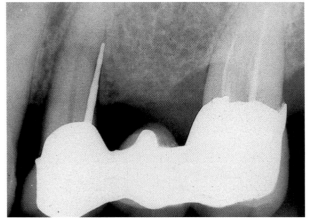

Fig 83

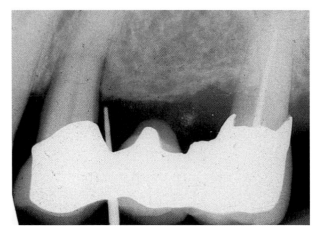

Fig 84

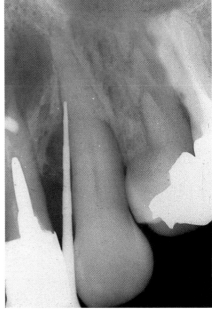

Fig 85

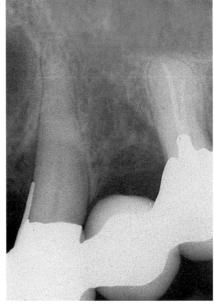

Fig 86

Figs 81 to 86 Use of matrix-guided material (Emdogain gel) on one- and two-wall bony defects.

Fig 81 One- and two-wall defects are visible along the distal surface of the right mandibular canine before treatment.

Fig 82 After 11 months, considerable gain in periodontal support was achieved.

Figs 83 and 84 Alveolar bony defect before treatment (Fig 83) and the result 6 months later (Fig 84).

Fig 85 Advanced one- and two-wall bony defects before treatment.

Fig 86 Result 6 months after treatment.

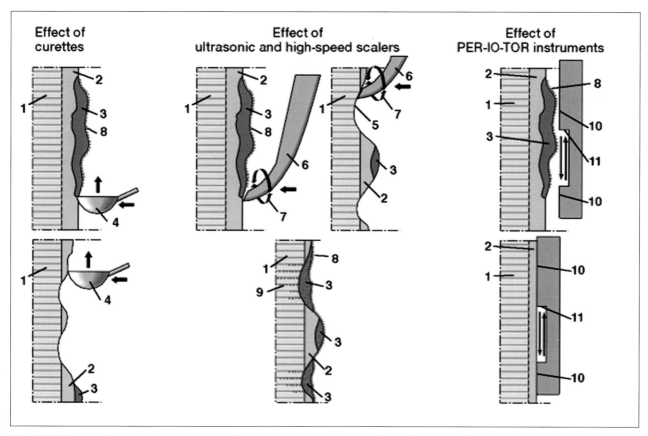

Fig 87 Difference between aggressive and nonaggressive instruments for scaling, root planing, and debridement: (1) root dentin with dentinal tubules; (2) root cementum; (3) calculus; (4) curette hand instrument; (5) iatrogenic rough, exposed dentin and dentinal tubules; (6, 7) ultrasonic or high-speed scaler; (8) subgingival plaque biofilm; (9) bacterial invasion of the dentinal tubules; (10, 11) principal design of reciprocating PER-IO-TOR instruments.

Fig 88 PER-IO-TOR nonaggressive reciprocating instruments (nos. 1 to 6). Different shapes and sizes facilitate access on concave and convex surfaces and furcation areas.

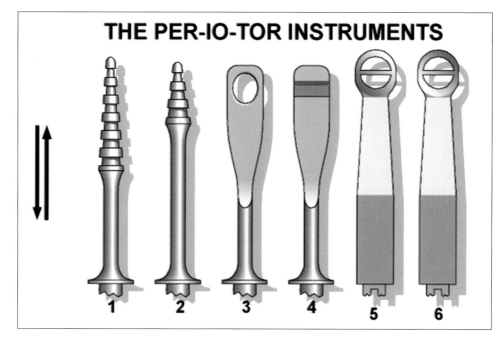

THE PER-IO-TOR INSTRUMENTS

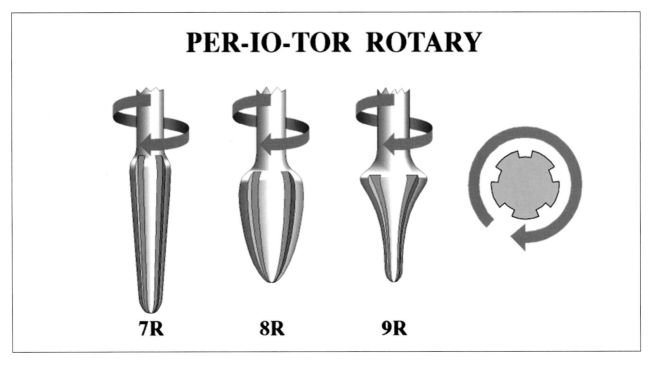

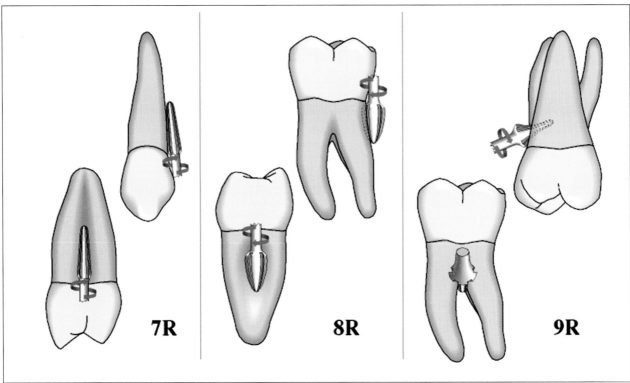

Figs 89 and 90 Rotating PER-IO-TOR instruments (nos. 7R, 8R, 9R).

CHEMICAL PLAQUE CONTROL

Chemical plaque control can be achieved through self-care or professionally. By far the most efficient plaque control programs are those combining mechanical and chemical methods: self-care, supplemented by needs-related PMTC and professional chemical plaque control (PCPC). For example, in mechanical plaque control through self-care, the toothpaste used usually contains not only an abrasive agent but also antiplaque or antimicrobial agents, such as sodium lauryl sulfate, stannous fluoride, triclosan plus zinc citrate, triclosan plus copolymers, triclosan plus pyrophosphate, or chlorhexidine digluconate (CHX).

Antiplaque and/or antimicrobial preparations (excluding antibiotics) suitable for self-care are available in a variety of vehicles, including toothpastes, mouthrinses, irrigants, gels, and chewing gums. For PCPC, several types of antiplaque and/or antimicrobial preparations are available, including pocket irrigants, gels, slow-release agents (varnishes), and controlled slow-release agents (Perio-chip).

Chemical plaque control should always be regarded as a needs-related supplement to, and not a substitute for, mechanical plaque control. Therefore, the choice of agent and frequency of use for self-care and professional care should be related to the individual patient's predicted risk for oral disease.

Self-care

1. Agents are applied with high frequency—one to three times per day, regularly or intermittently.
2. Accessibility and efficacy are good supragingivally, but very limited subgingivally and interproximally in the molar and premolar regions, particularly for mouthrinsing.
3. The method is compliance dependent and relatively costly for regular daily use, unless the agent is incorporated in toothpaste.

Professional chemical plaque control

1. The frequency should be needs related, and PCPC generally is more frequent during the initial intensive period to arrest enamel (incipient) caries, to convert active root caries to inactive, and to heal inflamed periodontal tissue as soon as possible and thereby reduce the Plaque Formation Rate Index (PFRI).
2. Accessibility is high because the agent is professionally applied.
3. The duration of effect can be extended by using slow-release agents, such as CHX-thymol varnish (Cervitec) and gels, and controlled slow-release agents, such as Perio-chip (CHX).

Goals of chemical plaque control

Chemical plaque control may be used for a variety of purposes:

1. To prevent plaque formation
2. To reduce the plaque formation rate (PFRI)
3. To control plaque formation
4. To reduce, disrupt, or remove existing plaque
5. To alter the composition of the plaque flora
6. To exert bactericidal or bacteriostatic effects on microflora implicated in caries and periodontal diseases
7. To alter the surface energy of the tooth and thereby reduce plaque adherence
8. To inhibit the release of virulence factors from plaque bacteria.

Although many antimicrobial agents would appear to be suitable for plaque control, few have demonstrated clinical efficacy, because of inherent problems in the mode of action of agents in the mouth and difficulties in incorporation in dental products. Although many of these agents exhibit broad-spectrum antimicrobial activity in the laboratory, they may display valuable selective properties on plaque.

The effect of an agent is concentration dependent. Initially, the inhibitor may briefly attain levels above the minimum inhibitory concentration, but subsequent desorption will reduce the concentrations. At sublethal levels, agents can effectively inhibit bacterial metabolism (eg, acid production and protease activity) and reduce the rate of bacterial growth. To increase antibacterial effectiveness, agents with complementary modes of action are being combined.

Long-term use of dental products containing antimicrobial agents must not (*1*) disrupt the natural balance of the oral microflora, (*2*) lead to colonization by exogenous organisms, or (*3*) lead to the development of microbial resistance. Several products that satisfy these criteria are now available and are clinically effective in helping to control plaque and gingivitis. As new agents and combinations of agents with improved antiplaque and antimicrobial properties are developed, the challenge will be to increase efficacy while preserving microbial homeostasis in the mouth.

Factors influencing the effects of chemical plaque control agents

Several factors influence the effects and bioavailability of different chemical plaque control agents, eg, substantivity, concentration, penetrability, selectivity, and delivery system.

Substantivity is defined as the ability of an agent to bind to tissue surfaces and be released over time, delivering an adequate dose of the active principal ingredient in the agent. Thus, the agent delivers the sustained activity necessary to confront bacteria attempting to colonize the tooth surfaces. The effect of a chemical plaque control agent is generally closely correlated with its *concentration*. *Penetrability* refers to the efficiency of an agent in penetrating deeply into the formed plaque matrix. The concept of *selectivity* implies that the agent has the ability to affect specific bacteria in a mixed population. Different *delivery systems* will in-

fluence the solubility, accessibility, and stability of the agent.

Solubility

Classically, an antiplaque agent must be solubilized in its delivery vehicle to allow rapid release into the oral environment, particularly when the application time is limited. The digluconate salt of chlorhexidine, for instance, was selected for the development of CHX mouthrinses on the basis of its high aqueous solubility. Triclosan, which has poor aqueous solubility, is solubilized in the flavor-surfactant phase of a dentifrice, facilitating its release and retention during application.

The bioactivity of an agent is not determined solely by its solubility. However, stabilizing an agent in solution may counteract its tendency to adsorb on the oral surfaces, because its chemical potential is reduced. This may occur for metal ions, for example, by complexation with ligands. Similarly, this may occur for sparingly soluble organic species by interaction with the surfactant or flavoring oils. The balance between solubility and stability in solution, on the one hand, and bioavailability, on the other, is a very important determinant of clinical benefit.

An alternative means of delivery is to deposit an antiplaque agent in the form of sparingly soluble particles within the oral cavity so that they deliver low doses of the agent over a long period. This principle has been used for slow-release devices, such as the antibiotic fibers used in the treatment of certain refractory cases of periodontitis, but has yet to be applied to antiplaque agents delivered from toothpastes.

Accessibility

Accessibility is critical for the effect of chemical plaque control agents and varies greatly for different delivery systems. For efficacy, the agent has to reach the site of action and be maintained at the site long enough to have a sustained effect. A study illustrating this point was conducted by Bouwsma et al (1992). Once-daily use of a wooden triangular interdental cleaner was more effective in reducing interdental bleeding than twice-daily rinsing with CHX, undoubtedly because the CHX rinse did not reach the interproximal site, whereas the mechanical interdental cleaning in the form of a wooden cleaner did.

These results are especially interesting in light of the observation that chemical agents are superior to physical agents designed for plaque removal, because chemical agents have a greater locus of activity as a result of their ability to diffuse into poorly accessible areas. However, in especially secluded areas of the oral cavity, such as the interproximal and subgingival areas, access is a prerequisite for diffusion to be effective. This suggests that local delivery of antimicrobial agents may have to be targeted to interproximal or subgingival areas. Reports of the efficacy of irrigators, supplemented with antimicrobial agents or not, demonstrated the importance of this approach in clinical management: Targeted delivery increases the efficacy of an agent, and random, nontargeted delivery of an otherwise potent drug can reduce its clinical benefits.

The pH and ionic interactions between an agent and receptor sites are important in determining the retention of a number of antiplaque agents, because the pH of the delivery vehicle governs the state of ionization of both the agent and the receptor groups in the oral cavity.

Stability

The stability of the agent is also important. Chemical breakdown or modification of an antiplaque agent may occur during storage, particularly at elevated temperatures. This may be due to the intrinsic instability of the agent in the presence of other ingredients, such as water, abrasives, or surfactants. Modification of an agent may also occur in the oral cavity, because of metabolic breakdown by salivary or bacterial enzymes. In either case, inactivation of the agent and loss of clinical efficacy ensue.

Antiplaque effects

As described earlier, plaque formation may be prevented by chemical agents by one or more of the following principles: (1) inhibition of bacterial colonization, (2) inhibition of bacterial growth and metabolism, (3) disruption of mature plaque, and (4) modification of plaque biochemistry and ecology.

Antiplaque effects may be exerted by interference with bacterial adsorption processes, rather than by direct antimicrobial activity. Various approaches to modifying the surface characteristics of teeth, pellicle, and/or bacteria in order to reduce bacterial adhesion to the tooth surfaces have been explored. Surface-modifying agents include anionic polymers and substituted amino-alcohols. They have high spreading action and may adsorb to enamel, thus lowering the free energy of its surface. Agents with the ability to aggregate in saliva could also reduce bacterial colonization.

Most chemical plaque control agents used today are broad-spectrum antimicrobials that exert direct bactericidal or bacteriostatic effects. They bind to the bacterial membrane and interfere with normal membrane functions, such as transport. This disturbs bacterial metabolism and may kill the bacteria. Adsorption to the bacterial membranes may also lead to alterations in permeability, resulting in leakage of intracellular components, along with protein denaturation and coagulation of cytoplasm contents.

In theory, caries may be prevented by chemical agents that reduce or alter the metabolic activity of plaque bacteria. The immediate clinical benefit of such agents is, however, questionable. On the other hand, long-term suppression of microbial metabolism, even by low-potency antimicrobial agents, such as fluoride metal ions, glucan-synthesis inhibitors, and certain sugar substitutes (eg, xylitol), may affect plaque biochemistry and ecology, because bacteria show varying degrees of susceptibility to the various agents.

Delivery vehicles

Chemical plaque control agents may be delivered to the oral cavity by various vehicles. The vehicle of choice depends, first, on compatibility between the active agent and the constituents of the vehicle. For instance, the early fluoride toothpastes were ineffective because of the incompatibility of fluoride with the abrasive system. Second, the vehicle should provide optimal bioavailability of the agent at its site of action. Third, patient compliance is of major importance. Patient compliance is probably reduced with increasing frequency of dose, length, and complexity of the treatment. Therefore, chemical plaque control is most likely to succeed if the delivery vehicle does not require the establishment of new habits or if the treatment is independent of patient compliance.

Mouthrinses

Mouthrinses are the simplest vehicles for antiplaque agents, the most common being a water-alcohol mixture to which flavor, nonionic surfactant, and humectant are added to improve cosmetic properties. Most antiplaque agents are compatible with this vehicle, although, notably, stannous fluoride has a short shelf life in a mouthrinse because of loss of stannous ions by precipitation.

Gels

Dental gels have been used mainly as delivery vehicles for chlorhexidine and stannous fluoride. The most common gel is a simple thickened aqueous system containing humectant but neither abrasive nor foaming agents. As such, it is com-patible with most antiplaque agents. Gels are usually applied in standard or custom-made trays to provide close contact with the agent and its site of action, ie, the plaque-covered tooth surface.

Toothpastes

A typical toothpaste contains an abrasive and a surfactant, which, together, are intended to remove loosely bound material, including plaque, pellicle, and stains. In addition, flavor is added for mouth freshness and therapeutic agents, particularly fluoride, are added for anticaries efficacy.

To deliver an antiplaque agent effectively, a toothpaste must have additional properties without compromising these basic functions. The complex mixture of toothpaste components should be physically and chemically compatible with the antiplaque agent to give a product that is stable during storage.

Chewing gums and lozenges

The release of various chemical plaque control agents from chewing gums and lozenges has been evaluated. As with sustained-release devices and varnishes, the effect will depend on release of the agent from the gum during chewing or from the lozenges as they dissolve. The contact time will increase, but increased salivation will inevitably increase the clearance rate of the agent from the oral cavity. Nevertheless, further work on chewing gums and lozenges as vehicles is warranted. Such vehicles may represent effective and acceptable routes, particularly in patients with low toothbrushing compliance. For individuals with reduced salivation, stimulation of salivary secretion by chewing may relieve discomfort.

Irrigants

Vehicles for chemical plaque control agents for supragingival and subgingival irrigation are of a composition similar to that of mouthrinses. Special devices for high-pressure irrigation through cannulae are available.

Varnishes and controlled slow-release devices

Devices and varnishes for sustained release and controlled slow release of chemical plaque control agents such as CHX may provide long-term contact between the agent and its site of action. The effect will depend on the degree and rate of release of the agent from the vehicle. Recently CHX and CHX-thymol varnishes have been introduced and are very effective in reducing plaque formation as well as mutans streptococci. A device for controlled slow release of CHX (Perio-chip) in diseased periodontal pockets has also recently been introduced. New data are promising (Jeffcoat et al, 1998).

Classification

In the literature different classifications systems for chemical plaque control agents, such as first- and second-generation antimicrobial agents, have been presented. The difference between these two categories is that the first-generation agents appear to be effective in vitro but lack substantivity and thus are not as effective in vivo. On the other hand, the second-generation agents, of which chlorhexidine is the principal example, are substantive and effective in vivo.

The most recent trend is to group chemical plaque control agents as follows:

1. Cationic agents
2. Anionic agents
3. Nonionic agents
4. Other agents
5. Combination agents

Cationic agents

Cationic agents are generally more potent antimicrobials than anionic or nonionic agents, because they bind readily to the negatively charged bacterial surface. Cationic agents can interact with both gram-positive and gram-negative bacteria and, by virtue of their antimicrobial properties, reduce the number of viable bacteria on the tooth surfaces or reduce the pathogenicity of established dental plaque. This has been confirmed in numerous studies (For reviews, see Emilson 1994; Addy et al, 1994).

The following groups of cationic agents have been tested or used as chemical plaque control agents:

1. Bisbiquanide detergents: chlorhexidine and alexidine
2. Quaternary ammonium compounds: cetylpyridinium chloride, benzethonium chloride, and domiphon beomide
3. Heavy metal salts: copper, tin, and zinc
4. Pyrimidines: hexetidine
5. Herbal extracts: sanguinarine

Of these, CHX is by far the most efficient and frequently used agent, followed by heavy metal salt compounds, such as stannous fluoride and zinc citrate. Chlorhexidine is used in all kinds of delivery systems (mouthrinses, gels, toothpastes, irrigants, varnishes, and controlled slow-release agents).

Chlorhexidine is still the most efficient chemical antiplaque agent of all, and is regarded as the gold standard; it has served as a positive control in most of the recent studies on chemical plaque control. Chlorhexidine also has a specific effect on mutans streptococci. A disadvantage is brown staining of the teeth and the tongue after some weeks' use, particularly from mouthrinses. Therefore CHX is not generally acceptable for daily long-term use, except in the recently introduced toothpastes. On the other hand, CHX is frequently and successfully used intermittently for 2 to 3 weeks in self-care mouthrinses and gels and in irrigants, varnishes, and controlled slow-release devices by professionals.

Anionic agents

Sodium lauryl sulfate is the most frequently used anionic chemical plaque control agent. Sodium lauryl sulfate is the most frequently used detergent in toothpastes but is also used in mouthrinses.

Cationic agents are inactivated by anionic agents. Use of CHX mouthrinse is not recommended immediately after use of toothpastes containing anions such as sodium lauryl sulfate and monofluorophosphate.

Nonionic agents

The most successful and frequently used nonionic plaque control agents (triclosan and Listerine [Warner-Lambert]) both belong to the category of noncharged phenolic compounds:

1. Phenol
2. Thymol
3. Listerine (thymol, eucalyptol, menthol, and methyl salicylate)
4. Triclosan
5. 2-Phelyphenol
6. Hexyl resorcinol

Listerine (named after Lister, the father of the antiseptics) was tested for efficacy against oral bacteria as early as 1884 by the legendary W. D. Miller. Listerine mouthrinse has been used for more than 100 years by millions of consumers, particularly in the United States. Its effect on plaque and gingivitis, although well documented, is less potent than that of CHX (Axelsson and Lindhe, 1987).

Triclosan, currently incorporated in commercial toothpastes and mouthrinses, is now the most important chemical plaque control agent in oral hygiene products for self-care. However, its well-documented effect on plaque and gingivitis is less potent than that provided by CHX (Ramberg et al, 1995b). Like other phenolic compounds, both Listerine and triclosan have an antiflammatory effect. The substantivity of triclosan is limited. To increase the substantivity, it has to be combined with other compounds. The most successful combinations to date are with copolymer (Colgate) and with zinc citrate (Pepsodent). Both combinations are used in fluoride toothpastes. The former is also used in fluoride mouthrinses.

Other agents

Very few agents in this group have been used. To date, Delmopinol is the most promising. It should be regarded as a surface-modifying agent and belongs to the group of substituted amino-alcohol compounds. The antiplaque effect of mouthrinses containing Delmopinol has recently been documented (Elworthy et al, 1995). Different enzymes have also been tested in toothpastes and mouthrinses, but without any substantial antiplaque effect.

Combination agents

As mentioned earlier, plaque is a complex aggregation of various bacterial species. It is therefore unlikely that one single agent can be effective against the complete flora. Combining two or more agents with complementary inhibiting modes of action may enhance the efficacy and reduce adverse effects of chemical plaque control agents, offering promising prospects for new and more effective chemical plaque control agents. Examples of improvement by combinations of agents are heavy metal ions (Zn^{++}) plus CHX or sodium lauryl sulfate; triclosan plus copolymer or zinc citrate; and stannous fluoride plus amine fluoride.

Summary

In vivo, it is clear that physical removal of plaque is possible only where there is direct contact with a mechanical tool. Plaque located in pits and fissures, or subgingivally, is not reached by mechanical brushing and interproximal toothcleaning and thus remains unaltered. Although chemical plaque control agents appear to be capable of overcoming some of the shortcomings inherent to methods of mechanical intervention, several difficult questions still have to be addressed. First, what level of suppression of the flora is realistic and desirable in a plaque-laden environment? Furthermore, how can the drug gain entrance into protected domains, such as the tonsillar crypts or the subgingival spaces, potential regions for repopulating bacterial species? At this time, neither site-directed chemotherapy nor lethal doses appear to be possible in the oral cavity. Finally, is antimicrobial therapy targeted to specific bacteria an attainable or desirable goal for the future? Perhaps 20 of the 350 species resident in the oral cavity are associated with either caries or periodontal disease, but the remainder are either neutral or beneficial to the host. Although few of the overall flora have been implicated in disease, an approach that focuses on specific bacteria, while ecologically correct, must await a better understanding of the pathogenic effects that occur at the molecular level.

For optimal effect of chemical plaque control agents, existing well-organized supra- and subgingival biofilms must be mechanically eliminated or ruptured because of the limited penetrability and accessibility of these agents and their delivery systems (for example, mouthrinses, irrigations, and gels).

For better compliance and cost effectiveness, the strategy for chemical plaque control by self-care should be to optimize the use of safe, efficient toothpastes. For professional use, the strategy should be to optimize safe, efficient, slow-release and controlled slow-release agents and devices.

CHAPTER 7

OTHER CARIES-PREVENTIVE FACTORS

For prevention and control of dental caries, posteruptive (topical) use of fluorides should be ranked number two among preventive factors (after plaque control), because fluoride reduces the demineralizing effects of the organic acids (acid excrement) produced by the cariogenic bacteria in the dental plaque and accelerates remineralization after the acid attack. Fissure caries can be specifically prevented and controlled by the use of fluoride-containing fissure sealants during eruption of the molars.

In populations and individuals with a high prevalence of caries, poor standards of oral hygiene, and no exposure to fluoride, a restriction in frequency of intake of sticky, sugar-containing products would result in some decrease in caries incidence. Salivary stimulation is an important caries-preventive measure in caries-susceptible patients who have a reduced salivary flow.

FLUORIDES

Fluorides have unique external modifying effects on caries initiation and progression. However, a prerequisite for optimal effect is a combination of excellent mechanical and chemical plaque con-trol, targeting the cause of dental caries—the cariogenic plaque.

The caries-inhibiting effect of fluoride (F) has been known for more than 50 years. Following pioneering work by Dean and coworkers (1942), for 50 years it was generally believed that the major caries-preventive effect of fluoride was preeruptive. Recommendations for use were based on the assumption that incorporation of fluoride in the enamel apatite lattice would confer to the enamel a resistance to acid dissolution, ie, that a high intake of fluoride during tooth formation and mineralization would result in fluoride-rich enamel, with enduring resistance to dental caries.

Preventive measures based on this assumption included fluoridation of public water supplies to the 1 mg/L level, or supplying children with fluoride in tablet form, salt, or milk. This approach is no longer accepted. Epidemiologic studies showed that, even where the water supply is optimally fluoridated, the topical effect of fluoride on the tooth environment is important; for example, children with erupted permanent teeth who move to a region with fluoridated water experience reductions in caries incidence, to levels similar to those in children born in the fluoridated region (Murray, 1969). At the same time, there was an increasing recognition of caries as a disease resulting from an imbalance between processes of mineral loss and gain, rather than an irreversible process of demineralization (Murray, 1969).

More and more inconsistencies gradually emerged between the concept of enamel resistance and actual clinical and experimental observations. It became clear that a high fluoride content in the hard dental tissues was of less importance than a moderate increase in fluoride concentration in oral fluids (Øgaard et al, 1991). Modern concepts of the mechanism of action of fluoride emphasize a daily supply, to establish and maintain a significant concentration in saliva and plaque fluid and thereby control enamel dissolution.

There is general agreement today among scientists in the field of fluoride research that the caries-preventive and caries-controlling effects of fluorides are almost exclusively posteruptive, ie, topical. The vehicle may be drinking water, slow-release tablets, or specific topical agents, such as toothpastes, gels, or varnishes. Much current fluoride research is concerned with improving the efficacy of topical treatments, based on an understanding of the mechanisms underlying the cariostatic action of fluoride. Laboratory studies have shown that fluoride not only reduces the equilibrium solubility of enamel (more or less apatite) but also exerts a wide range of effects on calcium phosphate chemistry, including the kinetics of dissolution and precipitation. (For review, see Ten Cate and Featherstone, 1996.) Fluoride also affects bacterial metabolism, particularly acid production and acid tolerance. It has been shown that the formation of fluoride reservoirs, in the form of calcium fluoride (CaF_2) on the tooth surfaces and in the tooth environment, is of great importance (Øgaard et al, 1983).

Occurrence and intake

In biology, fluoride is usually classified as a trace element and belongs to the halogen group (fluorine, chlorine, iodine, bromine). In biologic materials, the concentration of fluoride is generally as low as a few parts per million or less. However, fluorides occur in the environment at far higher concentrations than so-called trace elements.

Fluoride enters the atmosphere by volcanic action and returns to the earth's surface by deposition as dust, rain, snow, or fog. Fluoride enters the hydrosphere by leaching from soil and mineral into groundwater and by entry with surface water.

Because of the small radius of the fluorine atom, its effective surface charge is greater than that of any other element. As a consequence, fluoride is the most electronegative and reactive of all the elements. Because it reacts promptly with its environment, it occurs rarely in the free or elemental state in nature but most frequently in the form of inorganic fluoride compounds. The most important fluoride-containing minerals are fluorspar (fluorite, CaF_2) and fluorapatite [$Ca_{10}F_2(PO_4)_6$; 6.3% F], which are widespread in many countries.

Normally the fluoride concentration in groundwater is limited to 0.2 to 2.0 ppm, but, for example in the United States and some African countries, fluoride concentrations greater than 60.0 ppm have been reported. By contrast, most surface water contain less than 0.1 ppm of fluoride. In rivers, it may range from 0.1 to 1.0 ppm. Seawater contains 1.2 to 1.4 ppm of fluoride, depending on the chlorinity. Concentrations may be altered locally by undersea volcanic activity. Most fluoride in water exists as free fluoride ions.

Intake of fluoride is mainly from drinking water and beverages. It is estimated that about 60% to 65% comes from such sources in regions with less than 0.3 mg F/L in the drinking water, and about 75% to 80% comes from these sources in regions with higher fluoride concentrations. Mineral water may contain 1.8 to 5.8 mg of fluoride/L.

Tea leaves are a particularly rich source of fluoride, most of which is rapidly released into tea infusions, within 5 to 10 minutes. The fluoride concentrations of brewed tea commonly range from 0.5 to 4.0 ppm. As would be anticipated, fluoride concentrations in tea made with fluoridated water are somewhat greater than in tea brewed in water with low fluoride content.

Fluoride intake from diet (including drinking water and beverages with less than 6.0 mg of F/L) and recommended use of fluoride-containing dental products such as toothpastes, mouthrinses, lozenges, and chewing gums will normally have no adverse effect on general health in young adults and adults. However, up to the age of 6 years, it is well known that a high intake of fluoride will result in visible fluorosis of the teeth. The maturation phase of the maxillary incisors occurs at 22 to 26 months of age, when susceptibility to fluorosis is greatest (Evans and Stam, 1991). To prevent the development of visible and esthetically disturbing fluorosis, fluoride intake in infants and preschool children should therefore be limited and controlled.

The intake of fluoride associated with the development of enamel fluorosis of the permanent teeth has been estimated to range from 40 to 100 μg/kg of body weight per day. Infants consuming formulas made from concentrated liquids, or powders diluted with water providing 1,000 μg of fluoride/L, are at risk of dental fluorosis. The fluoride-concentration will increase when water is boiled in Teflon-coated vessels.

Toxicology

Topical fluoride agents are safe and harmless if used strictly as directed. However, systemic intake must be limited, because fluoride is a toxic substance. Based on the very few known cases of accidental death in children attributed to ingestion of fluoride, it is concluded that death is likely to occur if a child ingests a fluoride dose in excess of 15 mg of F/kg of body weight. A dose as low as 5 mg of F/kg of body weight may be fatal for some children. Therefore, the *probable toxic dose*, defined as the threshold dose that could cause serious or life-threatening systemic signs and symptoms necessitating immediate emergency treatment and hospitalization, is 5 mg of F/kg of body weight.

It is essential that the fluoride concentrations in dental products be known to the persons who use them. It is even more important to know the amounts of fluoride contained in standard packaging (bottles of tablets, tubes of toothpaste, etc) as well as the amounts involved during routine usage and how these amounts relate to the probable toxic dose.

Preeruptive effects of fluoride on tooth formation

Positive effects

Although the caries-inhibiting effect of fluoride is predominantly (almost totally) posteruptive, some positive preeruptive effects can be inferred, eg, during eruption of the molars, a critical period for the initiation of fissure caries, because of the extremely high plaque reaccumulation rate, until the teeth reach occlusion. In teeth, as in all the mineralized tissues, fluoride levels tend to be greatest at the surface nearest the tissue fluid that supplies the fluoride; preeruptive accumulation is highest on the pulpal aspect of the dentin and the outer surface of the enamel. A much higher total fluoride concentration is found in the dentin because of endogenous fluoride supply from the vessels of pulp. The outer surface of the enamel will receive a "topical" supply of fluoride from the surrounding follicular fluid, explaining why fluoride concentrations decrease from the inner surface of the dentin and the outer surface of the enamel, respectively.

The concentration of fluoride is also higher in those parts of the enamel that are the first to develop and mature, ie, the incisal edges of the anterior teeth and the occlusal surfaces of the molars and premolars. These preeruptive effects of fluoride may reduce susceptibility to initiation of fissure caries in the molars during eruption and possibly around the approximal contact surfaces before secondary, posteruptive maturation is completed.

Negative effects

By far the best known preeruptive effect of excessive fluoride intake is fluorosis, first described by Black and McKay, in 1916, as "mottled enamel." They suggested that it could be related to the water supply in the endemic areas. When it was subsequently shown in humans and in experimental animals that mottled enamel was an effect of fluoride on enamel formation and maturation, the condition was termed *enamel fluorosis.*

As early as the early 1940s, Dean et al (1941, 1942) demonstrated a positive correlation between the fluoride-concentration in the drinking water and the prevalence and severity of fluorosis. Numerous studies have subsequently confirmed that the risk of developing fluorosis is strongly correlated to the regular intake of fluoride during tooth mineralization, particularly during the maturation phase of the enamel. Dean (1936) suggested classification of the dentition into one of seven categories, according to the degree of enamel changes (fluorosis), from 0 for normal enamel to 7 for severe fluorosis. Scores from 1 to 6 comprised the stages questionable, very mild, mild, moderate, and moderately severe. Later Dean (1942) combined moderately severe and severe into one score, namely severe, to include all enamel surfaces with any type of surface destruction, irrespective of degree. At the time it was not known that, histopathologically, the entire tooth surface is affected, even in the mildest forms of fluorosis, and the distinction between very mild and moderate fluorosis was based on the area of tooth surface involved.

From studies in which the histopathology of fluorosis in human teeth was related to the clini-

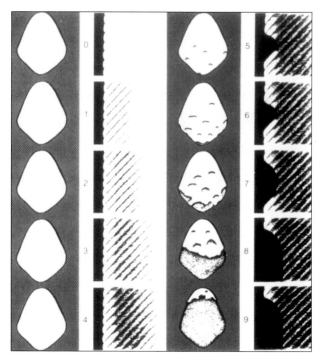

Fig 91 Thylstrup-Fejerskov Dental Fluorosis Index (1978). Scores range from 0 (normal) to 9 (most advanced form of fluorosis). The classification correlates clinical appearance and histopathologic changes. (Printed with permission from A. Thylstrup and O. Fejerskov.)

cal severity, Thylstrup and Fejerskov (1978) developed the so-called TF (Thylstrup-Fejerskov) Dental Fluorosis Index. Depending on the severity of the fluorosis, the enamel changes as observed on the single tooth surface can be arranged into 10 classes (Fig 91) scored from 0 (normal) to 9, for each degree of enamel change. To date, the TF Index is the only classification of fluorosis to correlate clinical appearance and histopathologic changes.

The risk for and severity of fluorosis are closely correlated with the plasma fluoride level during enamel maturation. The later in life enamel mineralization occurs, the more severe the enamel fluorosis is likely to be, even assuming a constant dose of fluoride from birth. The pattern of fluorosis in the permanent dentition is strongly correlated to the time of maturation of the tooth enamel for the homologous pairs of teeth.

Given the aforementioned association between the period of mineralization of the individual teeth and the severity of fluorosis, and assuming a constant exposure to fluoride, it is not surprising that dental fluorosis has seldom been reported in primary teeth. It was previously believed that fluorosis reflected excessive fluoride ingestion during the secretory phase of amelogenesis, but it is now known that the tooth continues to be vulnerable throughout the period of maturation.

Recent studies by Evans and Stam (1991) determined the relative risk of fluorosis of the central incisors because discoloration associated with fluorosis in these teeth is a serious esthetic problem. They found that the maxillary central incisors are most susceptible to fluorosis during the period of 22 to 26 months of age. For the incisors, fluoride exposure prior to this period carries less risk than exposure for up to 36 months subsequently; a period corresponding to the maturation phase of the incisors. The clinical implications are that central and lateral incisors are susceptible to fluorosis as a result of excessive fluoride intake up to age 5 years, with peak susceptibility at around the age of 2 years. Previously, it was believed that once the incisor crowns were complete radiographically, at about the age of 1 year, there was little or no further risk of fluorosis.

In the context of this new knowledge about the development of fluorosis and the fact that the caries-inhibiting effects of fluoride are almost exclusively posteruptive, there is no justification for systemic fluoride supplements (tablets). However, in children with a high risk of developing caries, slow-release fluoride-lozenges may be recommended for their posteruptive (topical) effect, once the permanent first molars begin to erupt.

Both water fluoride and tablet studies show that a daily intake of only 0.02 mg of F/kg of body weight during enamel maturation may result in fluorosis (prevalence, about 50%). The data also show that, even with very low intake from water, a certain level of fluorosis will be found. (For review, see Fejerskov et al, 1996.) In addition, the dose-response relationship is clearly linear; there is no critical value for fluoride intake, below which the effect on the enamel will not be manifested. Therefore, the conclusions of Hodge (1950), that dental fluorosis will not occur at a water fluoride concentration below 1.0 ppm, is no longer valid.

In this context, the administration of additional fluoride in tablet form to infants and small children in areas with water fluoride concentrations of less than 0.7 ppm will result in an increase in the prevalence and severity of fluorosis. It is surprising that such recommendations persist in some countries, particularly because of the extremely limited benefit of preeruptive administration. Also, the additive effect of ingestion from daily use of fluoride toothpaste (0.10% F) may increase the prevalence of fluorosis in areas with more than 0.2 to 0.3 ppm of fluoride in the drinking water. It is estimated that 2 to 3 year olds using fluoridated-toothpaste (0.10% F) twice a day will ingest about 0.04 mg of F/kg of body weight per day. Therefore, only a pea-sized amount of fluoridated toothpaste (0.10% to 0.15% F) is recommended for children aged 1 to 4 years.

Posteruptive effects of fluoride

For many years, the most important mode of action of fluoride was thought to be its incorporation into the apatite-like enamel crystals during development, resulting in crystals that were highly resistant to subsequent posteruptive acid attack. However, compared to the posteruptive effects, the preeruptive mode of action is now considered to be very minor.

Posteruptively, fluoride interferes with the carious process in various ways, such as inhibition of demineralization, enhancement of remineralization, reduction of acid production in the plaque, and reduction of plaque adhesiveness; the most important cariostatic role is in the aqueous phase on the tooth surface and between the enamel crystals during demineralization and remineralization.

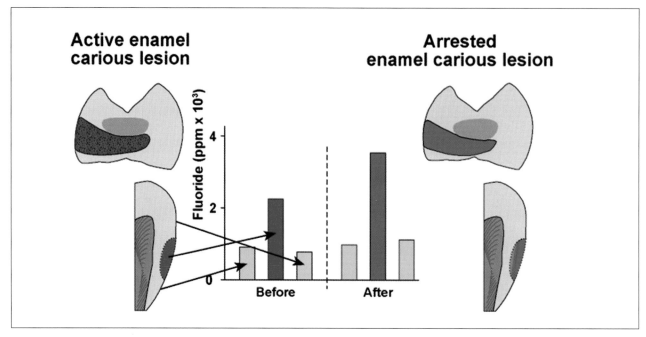

Fig 92 (left) Active, noncavitated enamel carious lesion on the mesiolingual surface of a mandibular second molar. (right) Lesion arrested by plaque control and administration of topical fluorides. (Modified from Wetherell et al, 1977).

Figure 92 shows an active, noncavitated enamel lesion on the mesiolingual surface of a mandibular second molar. Fluoride accumulates in the plaque fluid and, as CaF_2, on the enamel surface. During the acid challenge, CaF_2 is dissolved. The enamel surface acts as a "micropore filter," and F^- and H^+ ions (HF) diffuse into the subsurface lesion, increasing the amounts of fluoride in the active lesion compared to the surrounding intact enamel. Within the lesion, the F^- ions retard demineralization of the enamel crystals during the acid challenge and enhance remineralization by crystal growth and accumulation of fluorapatite (FA) on the crystal surfaces when the pH rises.

Such a lesion can successfully be arrested if the patient maintains a high standard of approximal plaque control and applies fluoride toothpaste (see Fig 92). Remineralization of the lesion is usually incomplete. "Continuous" access to a low concentration of fluoride results in more complete remineralization than a high concentration of fluoride, which induces more rapid remineraliza-

tion of the outer surface of the lesion (sealing the "micropore filter"). As a result, the remineralized enamel surface will be less caries prone than the original intact surface. The total amount of fluoride is increased in the arrested lesion (see Fig 92). These and other cariostatic effects of fluoride will be considered.

At the subclinical, microscopic level, repeated cycles of acid challenge, followed by a pH rise, combined with frequent (daily) access to low concentrations of fluoride from water and toothpaste, etc, will result in so-called secondary maturation, and the tooth enamel will gradually become more caries resistant. In vivo studies on the development of experimental carieslike lesions have shown that, in extracted unerupted teeth with mature enamel, the depth of the induced lesions is about one and a half, two, and three times greater than in extracted teeth exposed to the oral environment for 0 to 3 years, 4 to 10 years, and more than 30 years, respectively (Kotsanos and Darling, 1991).

Fig 93 Development of enamel caries. (Modified from Fejerskov and Clarkson, 1996.)

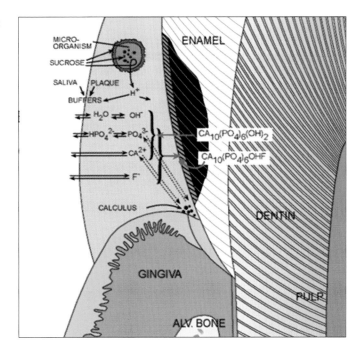

Dissolution of enamel

The physicochemical integrity of dental enamel in the oral environment is entirely dependent on the composition and chemical behavior of the surrounding fluids (saliva and plaque fluids). The main factors governing the stability of enamel apatite are pH and the free active concentrations of calcium, phosphate, and fluoride in solution.

The development of a clinical carious lesion involves a complicated interplay between a number of factors in the oral environment and the dental hard tissues. A simplified explanatory model of the major events is illustrated in Fig 93, modified from Fejerskov and Clarkson (1996). The carious process is initiated by bacterial fermentation of carbohydrates, leading to the formation of a variety of organic acids and a fall in pH. Initially, H^+ will be taken up by buffers in plaque and saliva, but, when the pH continues to fall (H^+ increases), the fluid medium will be depleted of OH^- and PO_3^{4+}, which react with H^+ to form H_2O and HPO_2^4. On total depletion, the pH can fall below the critical value of 5.5, where the aqueous phase becomes undersaturated with respect to hydroxyapatite. Therefore, whenever surface enamel is covered by a microbial deposit, the ongoing meta-bolic processes within this biomass result in pH fluctuations, and occasional steep drops in pH, which may result in dissolution of the mineralized surface.

Dissolution of enamel can result in the development of either a carious lesion or erosion. *Caries* is defined as the result of chemical dissolution of the dental hard tissues that is caused by bacterial degradation products, ie, acids produced by bacterial metabolism of low–molecular weight sugars in the diet. The *erosive lesion* is defined as chemical dissolution of tooth substance that is caused by any other acid-containing agent. Mixed lesions may well exist, particularly when the dentin has been exposed by erosion, causing hypersensitivity, which may lead to inadequate plaque control and caries. This condition occurs frequently on exposed root surfaces.

The appearance of the two lesions differs: the carious lesion is characterized by a subsurface demineralized lesion body, covered by a rather well-mineralized surface layer (see Figs 92 and 93). In erosion, the surface has been etched away layer by layer. No subsurface demineralization can be seen in the erosive lesion (Fig 94).

In principle, dental enamel can be dissolved under two different chemical conditions. When

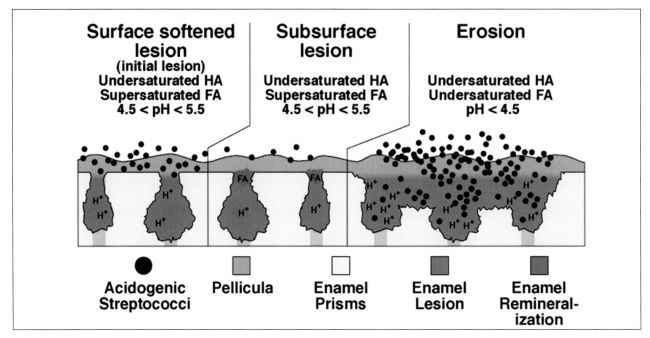

Fig 94 Mechanisms of enamel dissolution.

the surrounding aqueous phase is unsaturated with respect to hydroxyapatite (HA) and supersaturated with respect to fluorapatite, HA dissolves and FA is formed. The resulting lesion is a carious lesion in which the dissolving HA originates from subsurface enamel and FA is formed in the surface enamel layers. The higher the supersaturation with respect to FA, the more fluoride is taken up in the enamel surface, the better mineralized the surface enamel layer becomes, and the less demineralized is the subsurface body of the lesion.

On the other hand, if there is undersaturation with respect to both HA and FA, both apatites dissolve concurrently, and layer after layer is removed. This will result in an erosive lesion. Fresh acidic fruit, fruit juices, acidic carbonated soft drinks, and some champagnes are all unsaturated with respect to both apatites and are able to cause erosive demineralization of the teeth.

Progression of caries, from ultrastructural changes to visible decay, should be regarded as the cumulative effect of a long-alternating series of dissolution at low pH and partial reprecipita-

tion when pH rises. Eventually, after months or years, depending on the cariogenic challenge of the plaque, a clinically detectable white-spot lesion appears in the enamel.

Arrest of caries

Fluoride has a strong affinity for apatite, because of its small ionic size and strongly electronegative character. Two kinds of fluoride-apatite interaction occur: incorporation into the crystal lattice and binding to crystal surfaces. Both interactions have important consequences for the solubility and dissolution properties of apatite. The rate at which carious lesions progress is clearly heavily dependent on the rate at which the apatite crystals dissolve. It has been shown that the dissolution rate can be reduced by fluoride even without any reduction in solubility of the bulk mineral. This effect is the basis for topical fluoride treatments.

The presence of dissolved fluoride at concentrations as low as 0.5 mg/L in acidic solutions caus-

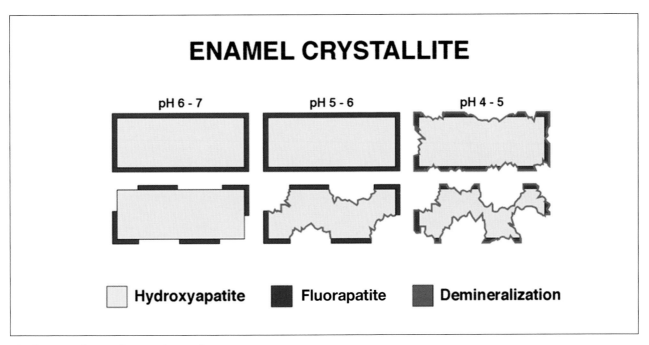

Fig 95 Dissolution of enamel crystallite.

es a reduction in the dissolution rate of initially fluoride-free apatite. Furthermore, pretreatment of apatite crystallites with fluoride solutions significantly reduces the susceptibility of the apatite to acid dissolution. These two effects are both the results of uptake of fluoride by the surfaces of the apatite crystals. Two types of uptake have been considered. In nonspecific binding, F- ions are adsorbed to the crystal surface without reacting chemically with it. In specific binding, ion exchange is involved, so that F- ions become incorporated into the crystal surface. The effect of surface fluoridation of the crystallites on dissolution depends on the proportion of the surface converted, because it appears that the nonfluoridated and fluoridated surfaces dissolve independently.

During a cariogenic challenge, both the concentration of fluoride at the crystal surfaces and the fluoride concentration in the liquid phase are important. To reduce the dissolution rate, fluoridation of the crystal surfaces, by whatever means, is necessary, but the surface fluoridation will be maintained only if the solution bathing the crys-

tals contains enough fluoride; otherwise, all parts of the crystal surfaces will dissolve (Fig 95).

Recently, the important cariostatic role of CaF_2 reservoirs on the tooth surfaces has been documented (Øgaard et al, 1992). Calcium fluoride globules, covered by a phosphate- and protein-rich layer, are formed (Fig 96). At neutral pH, CaF_2 precipitation at apatite crystals and on the surface of the enamel can be induced by application of dissolved fluoride at high concentration.

Because of its slow dissolution and hence prolonged retention, the solid CaF_2 is assumed to act as a reservoir for fluoride to be released into the liquid environment of the teeth (Fig 97). When all calcium fluoride is dissolved its effect is lost, and the calcium fluoride depot has to be replenished by repeated application of fluoride.

Formation of CaF_2 is possible at fluoride concentrations higher than 100 ppm, and the amount increases with increasing fluoride activity, prolonged exposure, and lower pH in the solution. Thus, significantly greater amounts of CaF_2 are precipitated after a 4-minute application of a 2% sodium fluoride (NaF) solution than

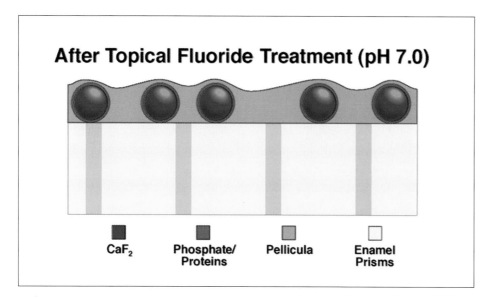

Fig 96 Tooth surface after topical fluoride treatment (pH 7.0).

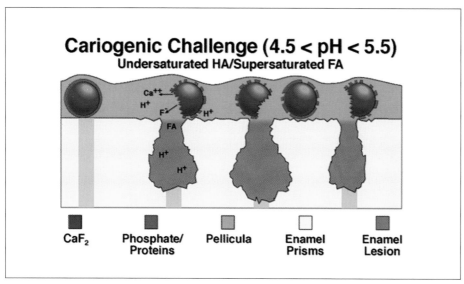

Fig 97 Tooth surface during cariogenic challenge (4.5 > pH < 5.5).

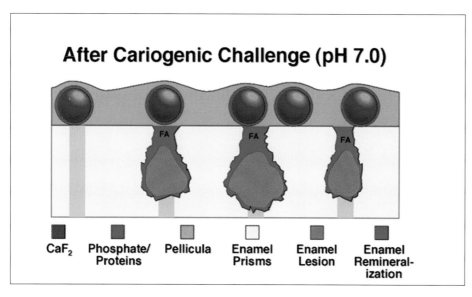

Fig 98 Tooth surface after cariogenic challenge (pH 7.0).

after a 2-minute mouthrinse with a 0.2% solution, and CaF_2 formation is considerably increased after use of an acidulated phosphate fluoride solution, because of the enhanced availability of calcium ions dissolved from the dental apatite. Modest amounts of CaF_2 may be formed from the use of NaF dentifrices. In contrast, extremely high amounts of CaF_2 may be expected from slow-release fluoride varnishes with high fluoride concentration; for example, a recently developed varnish contains 6% NaF and 6% CaF_2 (Bifluorid 12).

The dissolution of the CaF_2 seems to be the key to its caries-preventing effect, because only the free fluoride ion has an effect on enamel solubility. The dissolution of the CaF_2 globules covered with phosphate and proteins increases with decreased pH (see Fig 97), so that more ionic fluoride can be expected to be released during a cariogenic challenge. Fluoride ions will react with hydrogen ions as well as diffuse into the carious lesion, thereby slowing down the progression rate. However, this mechanism also implies that the CaF_2 reservoir will be depleted more rapidly in patients with high levels of carious activity. Therefore, efficient plaque control has to be introduced to increase the pH to 7.0 (clean teeth never decay), and this must be combined with frequent reapplication of fluoride. Thereby the enamel caries lesion will be arrested and the surface of the lesion remineralized with FA (Fig 98).

After topical application of concentrated fluorides, considerably more CaF_2 is formed in the micropores of carious lesions than on sound enamel surfaces (see Figs 92 and 98). The modest amounts produced on sound enamel surfaces can be expected to be lost within a relatively short period, ie, a few weeks, because of continuous exposure to physical forces, such as toothbrushing, and chemicals in food and beverages. In the less accessible micropores of the early carious lesion, however, CaF_2 may persist for prolonged periods, ie, months, strategically providing elevated fluoride levels at just the sites where the risk of carious progression would be expected to be greatest. The precipitation of CaF_2 in early carious lesions, with subsequent release of fluoride, is therefore believed to be a key mechanism for the caries-reducing effect of concentrated topical fluoride agents such as acidulated phosphate fluoride gels and varnishes (1% to 2% F). (For review, see Petersson, 1993.)

Remineralization

Mineral deposition in enamel defects such as the carious lesion may result in replacement or partial replacement of the lost mineral and is therefore called *remineralization*. White-spot or carious lesion remineralization is a widely documented phenomenon. (For review, see Ten Cate and Featherstone, 1996.)

When the impact of fluoride on lesion remineralization is studied, a distinction should be made between the effects on the remineralizing fluid of high doses of fluoride of short duration, eg, topical application of acidulated phosphate fluoride gels and varnishes (1% to 2% F) or even fluoride dentifrices, and a continuous low concentration of fluoride, eg, fluoridated water, or the intervals between toothbrushing or fluoride mouthrinsing. During and after short-term fluoride treatment, large amounts of fluoride are adsorbed in the lesion.

Enamel carious lesions contain considerably higher amounts of fluoride than the surrounding intact enamel; the F^- ions have great affinity for demineralized regions, where free Ca^{2+} and PO_4^{3-} ions are available in abundance for "marriage." Frequently the F^- ion marries both the Ca^{2+} and PO_4^{3-} ions, forming FA, but the favorite "wife" is the Ca^{2+} ion, resulting in CaF_2 (see Fig 98). The union of F^-, Ca^{2+}, and PO_4^{3-} (FA) is more stable than the marriage between the F^- ion and the Ca^{2+} ion (CaF_2), because they divorce easily during cariogenic challenge (4.5 > pH < 5.5) (see Fig 97).

After cariogenic challenge at pH 7.0, these two marriages are very important for remineralization. These marriages (precipitation of FA and CaF_2) will be accelerated in the outermost region of the lesion (see Fig 98), drawing away many of

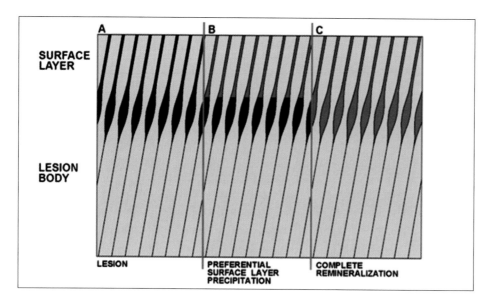

Fig 99 Development and arrest of an enamel lesion. (A) Active noncavitated enamel carious lesion. Observe the intraprismatic perforation of the surface "micropore filter" and the body lesion (black) beneath the surface. (B) short-term use of high-concentration fluoride; (C) long-term use of low-concentration fluoride. (Modified from Ten Cate and Featherstone, 1996.)

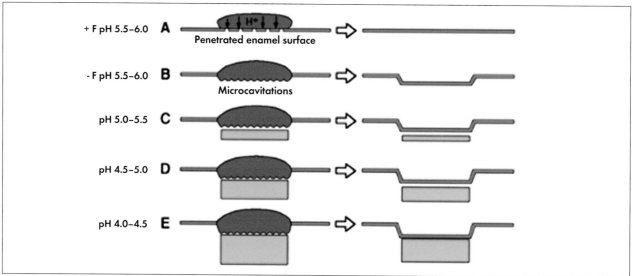

Fig 100 Arrest of carious lesions in enamel. (Modified from Thylstrup, 1994.)

the free mineral ions (wives) from the inner parts of the lesion (subsurface lesion or lesion body) and effectively slowing down diffusion toward the interior of the lesion. The result of high fluoride concentration is that demineralization in the lesion body is delayed and incomplete, compared to lesion formation in the presence of a very low fluoride concentration or in the absence of fluoride. Excess deposition of FA and CaF_2 may block the surface lesion pores, resulting in even more pronounced inhibition of diffusion.

Figure 99 (modified from Ten Cate and Featherstone, 1996) compares enamel lesion arrest after short-term use of high concentration fluoride to that after long-term use of low concentration fluoride. To date, the long-term effect of rapid arrest at the enamel surface has not been compared with a slow but more complete arrest throughout the entire enamel lesion.

Figure 100, modified from Thylstrup (1994), compares an active enamel carious lesion at moderate pH challenge, arrested by plaque control and topical fluoride, to active lesions at different pH challenges, arrested by plaque control without fluoride.

Topically applied fluoride

The posteruptive cariostatic effects of fluoride are correlated with fluoride concentration as well as with total exposure time. The latter is also influenced by the "substantivity" of fluoride in the oral cavity. For topical fluorides, such as dentifrices and mouthwashes, delivery of the fluoride to the site of action, and its subsequent retention, are as important for overall treatment efficacy as the chemical and biochemical interactions discussed earlier. This is partly because the treatments are applied for only a short period of time, often less than 1 minute, and partly because of subsequent washout by saliva.

Analysis of saliva after a single application of a fluoride dentifrice or mouthwash shows that much of the retained fluoride is cleared from the mouth within 1 hour. However, studies (Duckworth et al, 1991, 1994) also indicate a secondary clearance phase of 2 hours or more, during which the salivary fluoride concentration decreases more slowly. These authors postulated that the initial rapid clearance phase is the result of salivary washout and the second phase is initiated by the release into saliva of fluoride initially retained in oral reservoirs.

Potential reservoirs are the teeth, the plaque, the soft tissues of the gingiva, the tongue, the cheeks, and stagnation zones between the teeth, under the tongue, and in the buccal sulcus. The relative importance of the different sites is currently unclear. Plaque is important because of its proximity to the teeth. However, the soft tissues could be major reservoirs because of the relatively large surface area available.

The chemical nature of intraoral reservoirs may vary depending on the ecology (approximal surfaces of molars compared to lingual surfaces of mandibular incisors) and the topical fluoride agent used (fluoride-toothpaste [0.1%] compared to fluoride-varnish [> 2%]). From a cariostatic aspect, the most important fluoride reservoirs are, as mentioned, CaF_2 and fluoride bound to plaque bacteria. By far the most important effects of posteruptive (topical) use of fluoride are the inhibition of demineralization and enhancement of remineralization. Fluoride exerts physiochemical effects not only in the oral fluids, such as the interrod and intercrystalline fluid, pellicle fluid, plaque fluid, and saliva, but also bound in CaF_2, FA, and FHA (fluorohydroxyapatite).

However, fluoride also reduces acid formation in the dental plaque, may reduce plaque formation rate and plaque adhesion, and may change the ecology of the plaque microflora. Of these effects, the most important is the reduction of acid formation. The fall in plaque pH following sucrose exposure is reduced when plaque fluoride content has been enhanced by repeated topical treatment. However, it must again be emphasized that the most efficient way to prevent acid formation on the tooth surfaces is through frequent mechanical removal of cariogenic plaque supplemented by chemical plaque control to reduce plaque reaccumulation.

Fluoride alone is inadequate because its cariostatic effect is limited. If plaque pH falls below about 4.5, the plaque fluid becomes undersaturated with respect to fluorapatite, and demineralization will occur, regardless of the presence of fluoride. This is illustrated in Fig 101, modified from Kjaerheim (1995) (see also Figs 92 to 95 and 100). Human in situ experiments have shown that shark enamel, which consists of fluorapatite (33,000 ppm of fluoride), can be demineralized in the human oral environment within 1 month, when the specimens are covered by a 1-mm-thick layer of plaque biofilm. This also occurs in the presence of excess fluoride in the liquid phase above the enamel; ie, rinsing with fluoride does not prevent demineralization of shark enamel (Øgaard et al, 1991).

The oral hygiene of many patients at high risk for developing caries is inadequate. This probably causes the pH to fall to such a low level that even fluoride is unable to inhibit caries develop-

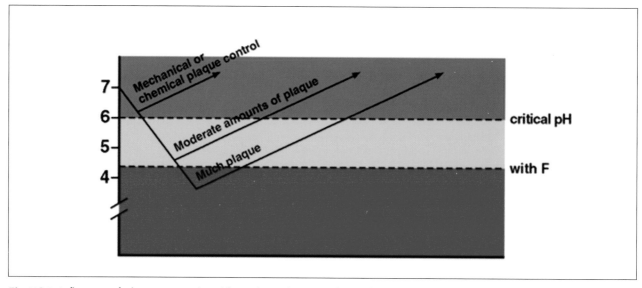

Fig 101 Influence of plaque control and fluoride on the critical pH of enamel. (Modified from Kjærheim, 1995.)

ment completely. In such cases, oral hygiene has to be improved, or fluoride administration must be supplemented by antibacterial agents, which prevent the pH from falling to a level at which fluorapatite dissolves (see Fig 101).

Systemically administered fluoride

As discussed already, the cariostatic effect of fluoride is almost 100% posteruptive. In other words, the caries reduction that has been achieved in studies based on systemic administration of fluoride should be regarded as a posteruptive (topical) effect of fluoride.

To date, fluoride has been systemically administered in drinking water, salt, milk, tablets, lozenges, chewing gums, and drops. Different concentrations of sodium fluoride have been used in these delivery systems.

Fluoridated drinking water is by far the most cost-effective public health measure for prevention and control of caries and reversal of subclinical lesions. This is attributable to the fact that, because most people drink water several times a day, even those without regular dental care and regular use of fluoride toothpaste benefit from water

fluoridation. Water fluoridation should therefore be recommended in all populations in which there is a relatively high caries prevalence, poor oral hygiene, and a lack of organized preventive programs or daily use of fluoride toothpaste.

A major obstacle may be lack of a reliable and controllable water supply, ie, centralized reticulation, in some developing countries or in rural areas of industrialized countries. The supply of fluoride from other sources must be known, in order to adjust water fluoride levels appropriately to reduce the risk of dental fluorosis. The recommended fluoride concentration in temperate climates, such as the United States, is 0.7 to 1.2 mg of F/L, but in warm to hot subtropical and tropical regions, only 0.5 to 0.7 mg of F/L is recommended, to prevent the development of esthetically unacceptable fluorosis.

Results from early studies with fluoridated water showed about 50% caries reduction in the permanent dentition and 40% in the primary dentition, compared to control areas. Significant reductions in root caries were also seen. (For review, see Murray et al, 1991.) At that time, caries prevalence was high in the United States and in Europe, where the studies were run, and few topical agents such as toothpaste and mouthrinses were available.

Nowadays, the supplementary effect of fluoridated drinking water would be only 5% to 25% in most European countries and the United States, because of improved oral hygiene and daily use of fluoride toothpaste and other topical fluoride agents, which have resulted in very significant reductions in both caries prevalence and incidence. However, in regions with relatively high caries prevalence, limited dental resources, and no daily use of fluoride toothpaste, water fluoridation should still achieve about 50% caries reduction.

However, only about 3% of the world population has access to fluoridated drinking water, mostly in the United States, where caries prevalence is low and almost 100% of the population use fluoride toothpaste and other topical fluoride agents daily. The use of the other fluoride delivery systems in the world is marginal (salt, 0.6%; tablets, etc, 0.3%). The current trend is toward a reduction in the use of fluoridated milk and salt and an increase in the use of fluoride lozenges and chewing gums, eg, in caries-susceptible adults with reduced salivary secretion rates.

The aim of using fluoride tablets is to achieve a supplementary posteruptive cariostatic effect similar to that provided by other topical fluoride agents, such as toothpaste. Therefore, only slow-release lozenges should be recommended, because of the prolonged fluoride clearance time in the oral fluids. An optimal effect should be achieved if the lozenges are used as a "dessert," directly after meals, particularly in adults with reduced salivary secretion rates.

To reduce the risk of fluorosis, fluoride tablets should not be used before the age of 5 years and absolutely not before the age of 3 years. Another problem with administration of fluoride tablets in public dental health programs for children is the limited compliance.

For very caries-susceptible patients, fluoride chewing gum should be the preferred systemic agent, to be used for 15 minutes directly after every meal. It is recommended primarily for caries-susceptible adults with reduced salivary secretion rates and for caries-susceptible children and young adults, especially during the eruption of the molars (5.5 to 7 years and 11.5 to 13 years).

The indications for fluoridated salt are limited, despite promising cariostatic results from controlled early studies in countries where the majority of the population does not use fluoride toothpaste daily (Colombia and Hungary) (Gillespie et al, 1985). With our current understanding of the cariostatic effects of fluoride, fluoridated salt should be restricted to populations in disadvantaged regions in the tropics and subtropics, where caries prevalence is relatively high and water fluoridation is not feasible.

There is only limited documentation available on fluoridated milk, and indications for its use are restricted because of the very limited topical effect (Stephan et al, 1984). If used at all, it should be restricted to daily use in elementary schools, when the permanent teeth are erupting or newly erupted, ie, in 6 to 13 year olds, in regions where fluoridated toothpaste is not used daily and fluoride mouthrinse programs cannot be organized.

Fluoride agents and compounds for topical use

Topical fluoride application is, without doubt, the most important means of fluoride administration for caries prevention and control. In particular, the widespread use of fluoride-containing toothpaste in conjunction with improved oral hygiene is thought to be the major factor contributing to the decrease in dental caries in those populations where it has been commonly used. As discussed earlier in this chapter, there is overwhelming scientific evidence that fluoride exerts its major cariostatic effect at the plaque-saliva-tooth interface during periods of caries dissolution and arrest. This also implies that the concentration of fluoride in a topical application or in the dental hard tissues is not, per se, an important determinant of cariostatic effect. These findings have thrown new light on the understanding and interpretation of results from different modes of topical fluoride applications.

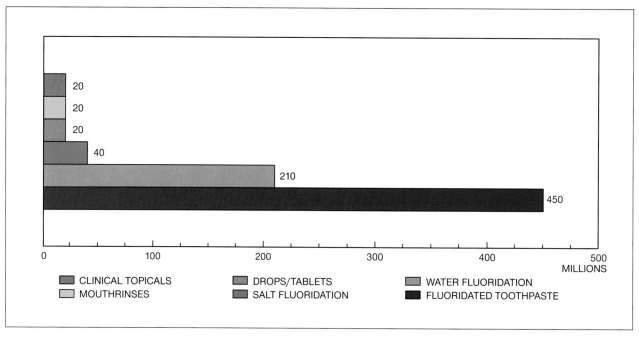

Fig 102 Estimate of the numbers of people in the world using various types of fluoride therapy. (Modified from the World Health Organization, 1994.)

Innumerable clinical studies on the caries-preventive effect of topical fluorides have been conducted over the past decades. The subjects, usually children and young adults, are often highly caries active and living in areas without water fluoridation. The duration of some studies has been several years, but the results of other studies have been presented after less than 1 year. The control groups are placebo groups or positive control groups exposed to another well-established fluoride caries-preventive measure. The diagnostic level at which caries is recorded, clinically and in some studies radiographically, has varied considerably between studies. Moreover, the design of the studies is often inadequate. Despite these confounding factors, overall the studies have shown the caries-preventive effect of most topical fluoride measures to range between 20% and 40%.

Topical fluoride agents are available for self-care or professional application (eg, by dentists, dental hygienists, or dental assistants). For self-care, the following fluoride agents can be used: toothpastes; toothpicks, dental tape, and dental floss; mouthrinses; gels, artificial saliva, lozenges, and chewing gum. Professionally applied fluoride agents are paints; gels; prophylaxis pastes; varnish, glass-ionomer cement (GC), and other slow-release agents.

Fluoride toothpaste is by far the most frequently used topical fluoride agent, used by 450 million people (Fig 102). Only 20 million people use mouthrinses or tablets, while 20 million receive professional applications of fluoride. However, although 450 million people use fluoride toothpaste regularly, more than 90% of the world's population does not have access to topical fluoride agents.

Many different fluoride compounds are used in agents for self-care and professional application. The three main categories are:

1. Inorganic compounds, including NaF, stannous fluoride (SnF_2), ammonium fluoride (NH_4F), etc: The salts are readily soluble, providing free fluoride.
2. Monofluorophosphate-containing compounds, such as sodium monofluorophosphate (Na_2FPO_3): The fluoride is covalently bound in the FPO_3^{2-} ion and apparently requires hydrolysis to free the F^-.
3. Organic fluorides, such as amine fluoride, and silane fluorides.

Sometimes two or more of the above compounds are combined in the same topical fluoride agent. The fluoride concentration in agents for self-care, such as toothpastes and mouthrinses, varies from 0.012% to 0.15% fluoride, while up to 1% fluoride is used in gels.

The fluoride concentration in agents for professional application is usually much higher, ranging from about 0.7% to 6.0%, which, as discussed earlier, will promote precipitation of CaF_2 reservoirs.

Delivery systems for topical self-application of fluorides

The following topical fluoride agents are available for self-care: toothpastes; toothpicks, dental floss, and dental tape; mouthrinses; gels; artificial saliva; lozenges; and chewing gum. The posteruptive cariostatic effects of lozenges and chewing gums have been addressed earlier in this chapter.

Toothpastes

The cariostatic effect of fluoride toothpastes was recognized more than 30 years ago. At present more than 90% of toothpastes in the industrialized countries contain fluoride (almost 100% in Scandinavia, but less than 50% in Japan). Although it is estimated that more than 450 million people use fluoride toothpaste regularly (see Fig 102), this represents less than 10% of the world's population. In other words, there is a huge untapped market for the introduction of a public dental health program based on inexpensive, effective fluoride toothpastes combined with improved oral hygiene habits.

The main functions of toothpastes are to facilitate mechanical plaque removal by brushing and to serve as vehicles for active agents (fluorides, chemical plaque control agents, anticalculus agents, etc). Toothpaste formulations may contain the following ingredients:

1. Active agents:
   a. One fluoride compound or two in combination
   b. Agents that potentiate the fluoride effect
   c. Chemical plaque control agents
   d. Anticalculus agents
   e. Antimercury agents
   f. Buffer systems
2. Abrasive particles
3. Detergents
4. Flavoring agents, preservatives, coloring agents
5. Thickeners, agents to regulate viscosity
6. Water

The following fluoride compounds are used in toothpastes:

1. Inorganic fluorides
   a. Sodium fluoride (NaF)
   b. Sodium monofluorophosphate (Na_2FPO_3)
   c. Stannous fluoride (SnF_2)
   d. Potassium fluoride (KF)
   e. Aluminum fluoride (AlF_3)
2. Organic fluorides
   a. Amine fluoride (Hetaflur)
   b. Amine fluoride (Olaflur)
3. Combinations of fluorides
   a. Sodium fluoride + sodium monofluorophosphate
   b. Amine fluoride + stannous fluoride
   c. Amine fluoride + sodium fluoride

Sodium fluoride and sodium monofluorophosphate are by far the most common, followed by stannous fluoride and amine fluoride.

Almost all the NaF, SnF_2, and amine fluoride in toothpastes will be dissolved in the mouth during brushing, releasing optimal amounts of free F^- ions. On the other hand, Na_2FPO_3 initially releases fewer free F^- ions, but also supplies FPO_3^{2-} ions, which within about 1 hour, are broken down by phosphate enzymes in the mouth, releasing F^- ions.

From 1955 to 1985 the standard fluoride concentration in toothpastes was about 1,000 ppm of fluoride (0.1% F = 1 mg F/g toothpaste), supplied as 0.2% NaF, 0.76% Na_2FPO_3, SMFP and 0.4% SnF_2. A wide range of fluoride concentrations, from 0.025% to 0.28%, has been used. The cariostatic effect of fluoride toothpastes is dose related. However, European Union regulations limit the concentration of fluoride in toothpastes to a maximum of 0.15%. Although there are no available data from double-blind studies comparing NaF, Na_2FPO_3, SnF_2, and amine fluoride in the same study, there are no indications that the differences would be more than marginal. The average caries reduction achieved in various 2- to 3-year clinical studies is about 25% to 30% (Johnson, 1993; Volpe et al, 1993). However, the cumulative effect over a lifespan is estimated to be 50% or more.

The cariostatic effects of fluoride toothpastes are also related to accessibility and fluoride clearance in the oral fluids. Accessibility may be improved by:

1. Frequent mechanical removal of dental plaque, particularly on the approximal surfaces of the posterior teeth
2. Deliberate application of fluoride toothpaste to the posterior interdental spaces before approximal cleaning
3. Thorough swishing with the remaining toothpaste slurry after cleaning, followed only by one brief rinse with water

The following measures may prolong fluoride clearance time from the oral fluids:

1. Using as high a fluoride concentration as possible.
2. Increasing the daily frequency of fluoride toothpaste.
3. Using the toothpaste technique recommended above.
4. Filling the posterior interdental spaces with fluoride toothpaste after cleaning at bedtime. This method is especially recommended for high-risk adult caries patients.

To minimize ingestion and the risk of fluorosis, for children younger than 6 years old, a pea-sized (5-mm) amount of toothpaste containing 0.10% to 0.15% fluoride is recommended. This is particularly important in areas with 1 mg or more of fluoride in the drinking water.

Toothpastes containing fluoride as well as chemical plaque control agents should be recommended, particularly to caries-susceptible patients with high plaque formation rates (Plaque Formation Rate Index score 4 to 5), periodontitis, or gingivitis. To date, the following formulations have proved most successful:

1. Sodium fluoride + triclosan + copolymer + sodium lauryl sulfate (silica-based) (Colgate Total)
2. Sodium monofluorophosphate + triclosan + zinc citrate + sodium lauryl sulfate (silica-based) (Pepsodent Ultra)
3. Sodium fluoride + chlorhexidine + zinc lactate (silica-based) (Crest, Procter & Gamble)

Toothpastes containing SnF_2 or amine fluoride also have documented antiplaque effects. (For review, see Richards and Banting, 1996.) However, to date the cariostatic effect of the above formulations has not been compared in a double-blind clinical trial. Even more efficient formulations are currently under development: the combination of mechanical and chemical plaque control plus fluoride in the same self-care procedure is too appealing and cost effective not to be optimally investigated.

Other oral hygiene aids

Oral hygiene aids that not only mechanically remove plaque but also, at the same time, release fluoride to the most caries-susceptible tooth surfaces in the dentition, the approximal surfaces of the posterior teeth, would be most appropriate. In recent years, several brands of fluoridated toothpicks (TePe, Butler, Elmex, Jordan, etc) and dental tape and floss (Johnson & Johnson, Oral-B, Butler, Elmex, Jordan, etc) have been introduced commercially.

Although to date no longitudinal clinical trials have been conducted to evaluate the effect of these new products on approximal caries, some in situ studies show that at least the use of fluoridated wooden toothpicks will elevate the salivary fluoride concentration to levels comparable to and even higher than those achieved by fluoride mouthrinses or lozenges; interproximally, the fluoride concentration should be considerably higher. However, both fluoride concentration and fluoride release differ significantly among the various brands (Kashani et al, 1998).

To optimize the release of fluoride from wooden toothpicks, moistening them in saliva for a few seconds just before application is recommended. Because toothpicks offer optimal accessibility to the key-risk posterior approximal surfaces, wooden toothpicks impregnated with NaF plus chlorhexidine would be an appropriate aid for prevention and control of caries as well as gingivitis and periodontitis.

Mouthrinses

Weekly school-based mouthrinsing with 10-mL neutral 0.2% NaF solutions for 1 minute are still very cost effective for caries control in regions where water fluoride concentration is low, for populations with a high prevalence of caries, poor oral hygiene, and no daily use of fluoride toothpaste. As mentioned earlier, more than 90% of the world's population does not use fluoride toothpaste. On the other hand, in areas with very low caries prevalence, a uniformly high standard of oral hygiene, and daily use of fluoride toothpaste, the supplementary caries-inhibiting effect of a weekly fluoride mouthrinse is negligible and not cost effective.

Rinsing with 10 mL of fluoride solution (0.025% F) for 1 minute after every toothcleaning procedure is an efficient supplement for caries control in caries-susceptible patients. Fluoride mouthrinses containing chemical plaque control agents (triclosan + copolymer + sodium lauryl sulfate [Colgate Total], chlorhexidine, amine fluoride + SnF_2 [Meridol], etc) should have a greater cariostatic effect than pure neutral NaF solutions. However, in patients with high caries risk (C3) and particularly in those with impaired salivary function (hyposalivation—less than 0.7 mL of stimulated saliva per minute—xerostomia), the combined use of fluoride and chlorhexidine chewing gums (Fertin) as a dessert for 15 to 20 minutes after every meal is a much more efficient cariostatic alternative than fluoride mouthrinsing to supplement daily use of fluoride toothpaste.

Gels

As with other fluoride and chemical plaque control agents, the effect of fluoride gels is related to the concentration, time of application, accessibility, and other factors. Although not recommended as a public health measure for self-care, for selected adult patients with a high risk of caries (C2-C3), fluoride gels must be regarded as efficient cariostatic supplements to fluoride toothpaste for daily use. Most commercial fluoride gels for daily use by self-care contain about 0.5% fluoride in the form of neutral NaF, acidulated phosphate fluoride, SnF_2, or amine fluoride plus NaF. The last two also have documented antiplaque effects. A gel containing both NaF and chlorhexidine is available by prescription. To improve the effect of the gels, the recommended application time is 4 minutes or more, preferably applied in customized trays.

Artificial saliva

For patients with dry mouth (xerostomia), artificial saliva containing NaF is available to improve physical and subjective symptoms and reduce the risk of rampant caries in these extremely high-risk patients. However, in these patients, meticulous mechanical and chemical plaque control and combinations of the most efficient fluoride agents are also essential. Fluoridated artificial saliva is formulated either as a gel or as a spray; patient acceptance is generally higher for the spray, which is usually applied 20 to 30 times a day.

Delivery systems for professional topical application of fluorides

The following systems are available for professional application: fluoride solutions for painting, gels, prophylaxis pastes, and slow-release agents, such as varnishes and glass-ionomer cements. The fluoride concentration in agents for professional use is generally much higher than for self-care and normally ranges from 1% to 2%. The fluoride compounds most commonly used professionally are neutral NaF, acidulated phosphate fluoride, and SnF$_2$. Amine fluoride and silane fluoride are also used in some commercial products. For optimal accessibility, plaque must be removed by professional mechanical toothcleaning before the fluoride agent is applied to the tooth surfaces at greatest risk.

Professionally applied fluoride agents are no longer recommended for public health programs. Some exceptions may be the following: (*1*) for areas with relatively homogenous high-risk prevalence, fluoride-deficient drinking water and lack of fluoride toothpaste, but personnel resources available for a school-based preventive program; (*2*) in special risk groups such as the mentally handicapped or elderly people with reduced saliva flow, exposed root surfaces, and heavily restored dentitions; and (*3*) in people with senile dementia. From a cost-effectiveness aspect, pro-

fessionally applied fluoride agents are also justified as a public health measure for specific age groups of children, during eruption of the first and second molars (5 to 7 year olds and 11 to 13 year olds).

In populations in which caries prevalence is low and there is daily use of fluoride toothpaste and possibly fluoridated drinking water, the intervals and selection of fluoride agent for supplementary professional application should be based strictly on individual needs.

Fluoride solutions for painting

The most common fluoride solutions for painting are neutral 2% NaF (1% F), 8% SnF$_2$ (2% F) and acidulated phosphate fluoride (1.23% F). Amine fluoride solutions are also used. Although this method is uncommon nowadays, application of 8% SnF$_2$ to the root surfaces of patients susceptible to root caries can still be recommended as a relatively cost-effective method, because of the combined fluoride and antimicrobial effect.

Fluoride gels

Fluoride gels for professional use contain a similar assortment of fluoride compounds as gels for self-care, namely neutral NaF, acidulated phosphate fluoride, SnF$_2$, amine fluoride plus NaF, and, by prescription, NaF + chlorhexidine. For optimal accessibility, plaque must be removed by professional mechanical toothcleaning, the gel syringed into the posterior interproximal spaces, followed by gel application in a customized tray for more than 4 minutes. Fluoride gels are recommended for use at strictly needs-related intervals in selected patients at risk for developing caries (C2 or C3). Gels containing SnF$_2$, amine fluoride plus NaF, and particularly NaF + chlorhexidine have combined fluoride and antiplaque effects.

Prophylaxis pastes

Prophylaxis pastes are used mainly for professional mechanical toothcleaning but also for finishing and polishing. The abrasiveness is evaluated in radioactive dentin abrasivity (RDA) or dentin abrasive value (DAV). For polishing and professional mechanical toothcleaning on root surfaces and composite fillings RDA 40 to 90 should be used, while RDA 100 to 200 is recommended for regular professional mechanical toothcleaning and RDA greater than 200 is recommended for finishing. Although all prophylaxis pastes should contain fluoride, the fluoride effect should not be overestimated; in caries-susceptible patients, more efficient agents, such as fluoride varnishes, are recommended to supplement professional mechanical toothcleaning.

Semislow-release and slow-release fluoride agents

Semislow-release and slow-release fluoride agents, such as fluoride varnishes and glass-ionomer cements, are rapidly growing in popularity for professional use, because of the greater cost effectiveness of the slow release of fluoride.

Three major fluoride varnishes are commercially available: Duraphat (5% NaF; 2.3% F), Fluor Protector (silan fluoride; 0.1% F) and Bifluorid 12 (6% NaF + 6% CaF_2; about 6% F). Based on clinical studies, the caries reduction achieved by fluoride varnishes ranges from about 20% to 70% (Pettersson, 1993). To date, the three different fluoride varnishes have not been compared in a well-controlled longitudinal clinical study. Experimental studies indicate that Bifluorid 12 should be the most efficient, at least in reducing dentinal hypersensitivity (Schroers, 1994).

However, the caries-reducing effect of fluoride varnishes results from a combination of mechanical removal of plaque by professional mechanical toothcleaning, protection of the cleaned caries-susceptible tooth surfaces from direct contact with reaccumulated plaque, and slow release of fluoride, for as long as the varnish is retained. Therefore, it is recommended that the initial varnish application be repeated three times within 7 to 10 days in patients with caries risk, to heal gingivitis, thereby reducing the plaque formation rate, and to arrest enamel caries by sealing the outer micropore surface as soon as possible. Thereafter, the varnish should be reapplied at needs-related intervals, two to four times per year.

Two types of specific intraoral slow-release devices have been developed: the copolymer membrane device and the fluoride glass device. To date, no results have been presented from ongoing clinical studies in the United States and the United Kingdom.

The assortment of restorative materials, sealants, liners, and cements that contain fluoride and act as slow-release fluoride agents is continuously increasing. The pure glass-ionomer cements release significantly most fluoride, followed by resin-modified GCs, GC-modified resin composites (compomers) and fluoridated resin composites and amalgams.

In addition to the benefit of slow release of fluoride, particularly from GC materials, such materials can be "recharged" with fluoride from other sources, such as daily use of toothpastes, lozenges, and chewing gums. The fastest and most efficient method of recharging GC restorations and sealants with fluoride would be by application of fluoride varnish with a high fluoride concentration, such as Bifluorid 12 (6% NaF plus 6% CaF_2).

Experimental in situ as well as clinical studies have shown that GC is very efficient in preventing secondary caries in caries-susceptible patients (Ten Cate and Van Duinen, 1995; Seppä, 1994). In addition, low-viscosity GC is strongly recommended as a slow-release fluoride sealant in erupting molars. The practice of applying acid-etched resin composite sealants to the fissures of fully erupted caries-free molars should now be regarded as an outmoded, expensive overtreatment.

FISSURE SEALANTS

Data on the decline of caries prevalence among children and young adults in most industrialized countries over the last two decades show a relative increase in the proportion of caries on the occlusal surfaces of the permanent molars (Bratthall et al, 1996). Even in developing countries with relatively low caries prevalence, the occlusal surfaces of the permanent molars are decayed more frequently than the approximal surfaces.

Fissure caries is partly attributed to the extremely plaque-retentive morphology of the fissure systems. To prevent the accumulation of cariogenic plaque in the depths of the fissures, and thereby prevent the development of caries, so-called fissure sealants were introduced to level out the original occlusal morphology.

Indications

In the early 1970s, in Scandinavia, as in most industrialized countries, there were practically no unrestored occlusal surfaces of permanent first molars in 11- to 12-year-old children. This was because of the combined effect of a very high caries incidence and the universal application of G. V. Black's principle of "extension for prevention": Many caries-free fissures were "preventively sealed" with amalgam restorations.

In a 5-year longitudinal study, Månsson (1977) followed caries progression in the fissures of the permanent first molars from eruption. Despite the prevailing very high caries incidence in Sweden, only 50% of the occlusal surfaces decayed; ie, 100% successful use of fissure sealants would have resulted in a maximum caries reduction of 50%.

If restorative therapy were limited to caries with cavitation into dentin, at the current very low caries incidence, restorations would be indicated in only about 5% of the occlusal surfaces. Cavitation confined to the enamel would be managed by minimal intervention: so-called sealant restorations or fissure sealants. Widespread use of fissure sealants cannot be justified as cost effective in our population today, because 100% success will result in a caries reduction of only about 5%.

A study by Carvalho et al (1989) has shown that initiation of almost all fissure caries in the permanent molars occurs during the extremely long period of eruption (1.0 to 1.5 years, compared to only 1 to 2 months in premolars). This also explains why fissure caries seldom develops in premolars.

Particularly in the distal and central fossae with surrounding fissures, plaque reaccumulation is extremely high on the occlusal surfaces of erupting molars compared to fully erupted molars, where it is effectively limited by abrasion from normal mastication (Figs 103 and 104). (See also Fig 26.)

For cost effectiveness, plaque control and use of fluorides should therefore be intensified during the critical period of eruption and supplemented, in selected children with caries risk (C2) and high caries risk (C3), with fluoride-releasing fissure sealants. A general strategy of fissure sealing the occlusal surfaces of fully erupted caries-free molars must be regarded as expensive overtreatment.

A study of occlusal caries in erupting permanent first molars showed that a needs-related, non-invasive preventive program arrested or inactivated about 80% to 90% of active enamel lesions (Carvalho et al, 1992). After 3 years, only 2% of the occlusal surfaces had to be sealed, and none had to be restored. No progression of lesions into dentin was observed on bitewing radiographs. During the eruption of the molars, the parents were taught to clean the occlusal surfaces of their children's teeth with a specific toothbrushing technique and fluoride toothpaste. In selected children with higher caries risk (C2, C3), home care was supplemented, at needs-related intervals, by professional mechanical toothcleaning and application of 2% NaF solution. In a matched control group, despite massive use of topical fluoride and fissure sealing of 70%, 2% of the occlusal surfaces had to be restored (Carvalho et al, 1992).

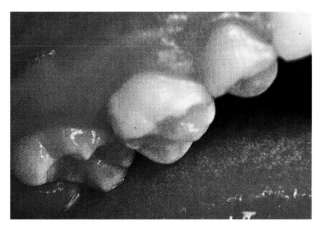

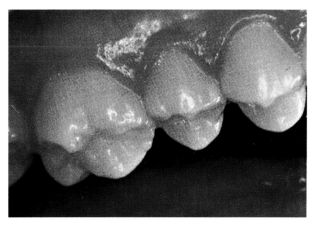

Fig 103 Plaque accumulation on the occlusal surfaces of partially erupted molars. (Courtesy of Dr A. Thylstrup.)

Fig 104 Plaque accumulation on the occlusal surfaces of the same molars, now completely erupted. (Courtesy of Dr A. Thylstrup.)

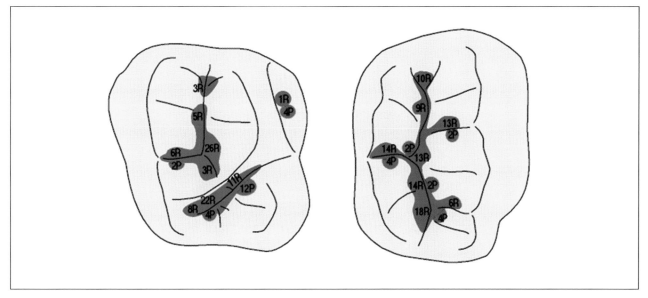

Fig 105 Development of occlusal enamel caries in children in a noninvasive preventive program. (green) Arrested caries; (red) enamel caries that has not progressed to cavitation. (Modified from Carvalho et al, 1992.)

In addition, in the test groups, many initially active carious lesions in enamel were arrested, and a few carious lesions in enamel developed but did not progress to cavitation (Fig 105). This low-cost, noninvasive program was subsequently implemented on a large scale, and over a 10-year period the percentage of caries free 12 year olds increased from about 30% to almost 90%, without the use of fissure sealants (Thylstrup et al, 1997).

However, in populations with high caries prevalence and incidence, the earliest possible use of fluoride-releasing fissure sealants in the permanent first and second molars is still a very efficient method of caries control.

Development

Successful sealing of occlusal fissures was first achieved in 1955 by Buonocore, who reported that treatment of enamel with phosphoric acid allowed resin materials to penetrate the microspaces of etched enamel. This acid-etch technique for enamel-retained modern dental resin materials (bis dimethacrylate [BDMA]) was introduced as the fissure sealant technique.

Commercially available sealants differ as to whether they are free of inert fillers or are semifilled and whether they are clear, tinted, or opaque. A major difference is the manner in which polymerization is initiated. The original (first-generation) sealants were activated by ultraviolet light. Second-generation sealants are autopolymerizing and set on mixing with a chemical catalyst-accelerator system. The third-generation sealants are photoinitiated by visible light. Another recent innovation is the availability of fluoride-containing sealants.

Recently, glass-ionomer cements (GCs) and resin-modified GCs have also been introduced as caries-preventive fissure sealants. These materials should not be regarded as semipermanent fissure sealants, but as efficient, slow-release fluoride agents, in which the depleted fluoride reservoir can be replenished from fluoride sources such as varnishes, gels, etc. Placement of GC would be more appropriate during eruption, when the fissures are most caries susceptible, even though most of the GC material is lost shortly after full eruption, by which time the risk of caries in these fissures is negligible (see Figs 26 and 103 to 105).

On the other hand, the second- and third-generation enamel-retained resin fissure sealants have been successful in fully erupted teeth. In a 10-year longitudinal study of second-generation sealants, Wendt and Koch (1988) reported a 70% to 95% success rate. In partially erupted teeth, the reported success rate has been only about 50% (For review, see Ripa, 1993.). The question arises as to how many surfaces, if left unsealed, would have developed carious lesions that progressed to cavitation.

Application

A major reason for the disappointing results in erupting teeth is that the acid-etching technique is very sensitive to salivary contamination: Retention of the fissure sealant depends almost entirely on the efficiency of the clinical moisture control. During the sealing procedure, the tooth must be kept completely dry. This is very difficult when the extremely caries-prone distal fossae in erupting molars are sealed. If the etched enamel is contaminated with saliva, the surface should be carefully rinsed with water and dried, and only after new moisture control procedures are followed should the etching be repeated. Otherwise "secondary caries" may be initiated in the gap between the etched enamel and the resin.

For etching, 30% phosphoric acid solutions or gels are generally used with resin-based sealants. The phosphoric acid treatment causes microscopic etching of enamel that allows resinous sealant materials to penetrate the enamel. The bond formed is purely mechanical.

Polyacrylic acid is used to prepare fissures for sealing with glass-ionomer cements. This procedure should be regarded as a chemical conditioning of the surface and not an etching treatment. The reaction between GC and the dental tissues is chemical, and the bond strength is considerably weaker than that achieved with the acid-etching technique.

Efficacy

In a 4-year study, the caries-preventive effect of resin-based fissure sealant (Delton) was compared with GC (Fuji III) (Mejáre and Mjör, 1990). The results showed that 100% of the occlusal surfaces sealed with GC were caries free, even though more than 60% of the material was lost within 6 to 12 months, and 95% was lost after 30 to 36 months. In the occlusal surfaces sealed with resin-based sealants, about 95% were caries free, and about 90% of the sealants were retained (for review of fissure sealants, see Ripa, 1993).

Type of fissure	Caries risk	Treatment	%
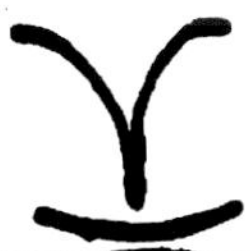	No or low	PMTC + F varnish	**70**
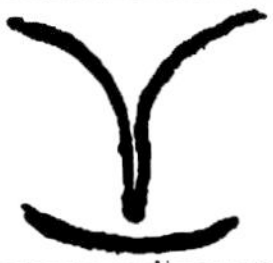	High or very high	PMTC + fissure sealant (glass-ionomer)	**10**
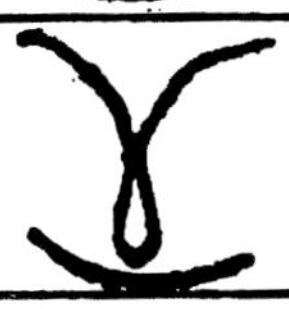	No or low	PMTC + fissure sealant (glass-ionomer)	**10**
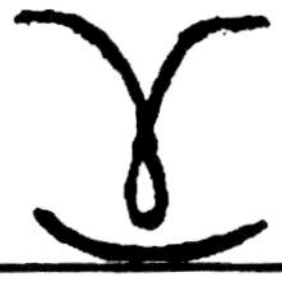	High or very high	PMTC + fissure sealant (glass-ionomer)	**10**

Fig 106 Preventive program for the occlusal surfaces of the molars, selected at the beginning of molar eruption. The aims are maintaining caries-free occlusal surfaces and, at the most, use of a fissure sealant or so-called "fissure blocking." (PMTC) Professional mechanical toothcleaning.

From a cost-effectiveness aspect, it can be concluded that the use of fissure sealants should be needs related and not a general procedure. On the basis of predicted caries risk and the anatomy of the fissures (Fig 106), erupting molars should be sealed as early as possible, preferably with a fluoride-releasing material.

DIETARY CONTROL

Sugar is not a causative factor in dental caries but an external modifying risk factor, as previously discussed. The objective of dietary evaluations and recommendations related to dental caries should be to reduce the total sugar clearance time per day. However, because root caries can develop at pH as high as 6, intake of sticky, starch-containing products must also be regarded as a powerful modifying factor in elderly people with exposed root surfaces and impaired salivary function.

High salivary levels of lactobacilli indicate a high sugar intake and low pH in the oral cavity. The lactobacillus test is useful as an objective supplement to the dietary questionnaire. Sugar intake can easily be assessed from a so-called 24-hour recall questionnaire or by using specially designed questionnaires for estimation of sugar clearance time.

For caries prevention and control, the following five dietary recommendations are realistic and essential:

1. Breakfast, the first meal of the day, should be a balanced composition of dairy products, grains, and fruit, eg, yogurt and muesli (fibers, cornflakes, etc), fresh fruit, and vegetables. This is in sharp contrast to the so-called continental breakfast, containing mainly sugar, fat, and water, which causes rapid swings in blood sugar levels, stimulating a high frequency of sugar intake all day.
2. The total daily number of meals, including between-meal snacks, should be limited to about

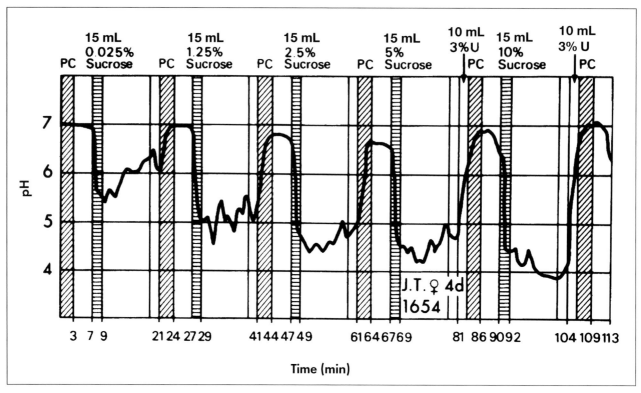

Fig 107 Drop in pH and sugar clearance time beneath 4-day-old (4d) undisturbed approximal plaque, evaluated in vivo by the Telemetric method. (Reprinted from Imfeld, 1978. Used with permission.)

four. This reduces total sugar clearance time and the number of drops in pH. Patients should be made aware that, within 5 minutes, even a very weak sucrose solution (5%) results in a fall in pH to suboptimal levels beneath 2- to 3-day-old plaque. Such conditions would apply to the approximal surfaces in a toothbrushing population (Fig 107).

3. Sticky, sugar-containing products, which result in prolonged sugar clearance times, should be eliminated (Fig 108). Sugarless sweets, containing sugar substitutes such as xylitol, sorbitol, saccharin, and aspartame, should be used.

4. In each meal, fiber-rich products that stimulate chewing and salivary flow should be included.

5. Selected individuals with high risk of developing caries (Plaque Formation Rate Index scores ranging between 3 and 5) and reduced salivary secretion rates should clean all tooth surfaces just before each meal, to limit the drop in pH during and immediately after the meal. Sugar-

less fluoride chewing gum (Fluorette, Dentan) or fluoride lozenges (Fludent, Dentan) are recommended after each meal as a dessert, not only to stimulate salivary flow but also to increase fluoride levels for remineralization after the acid attack.

SALIVARY STIMULATION

Reduced salivary flow is a very important internal modifying risk factor and prognostic risk factor for dental caries. Thus, salivary stimulation is very important in caries-susceptible patients with reduced salivary flow.

Many salivary stimulation materials and methods are available: Physiologically, saliva is stimulated by fiber-rich, well-flavored, aromatic food. The most attractive salivary stimulation agents for

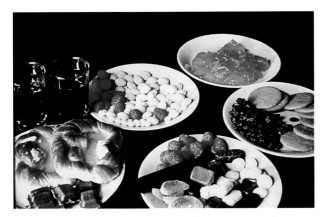

Fig 108 Sticky, sugar-containing foods that result in prolonged sugar clearance times.

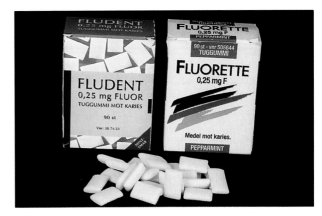

Fig 109 Sugarless fluoridated chewing gums.

caries prevention are the recently introduced commercially available sugarless fluoride chewing gums, Fluorette and Fludent (Fig 109), recommended as a dessert, to be chewed for 15 to 20 minutes, directly after every meal. In a 6-month longitudinal study on a selected group of caries-susceptible adults with very low salivary flow rates, use of fluoride chewing gum for 15 minutes after every meal increased the stimulated salivary secretion rate by 50% (Axelsson et al, 1997). Salivary mutans streptococci was considerably reduced, and the Plaque Formation Rate Index decreased by 30%.

A chewing gum containing chlorhexidine (Fertin) has also recently been introduced. Combining fluoride and chlorhexidine chewing gums would not only improve salivary stimulation but also prolong fluoride clearance time and provide chemical plaque control directly after the acid attack. Fluoride lozenges (Fludent or Dentan), used at the same needs-related intervals, are an alternative to sugarless fluoride chewing gums.

Tablets made specifically to stimulate salivary flow are also commercially available. These tablets, such as the Swedish SST (Salivary Stimulating Tablet), and Salivin, contain malic acid (from fruit). The SST contains a special buffer system to prevent erosion and has been tested daily for 6 months, without side effects.

To reduce subjective symptoms in xerostomia patients, fluoride-containing artificial saliva is available in spray form; patient acceptance is high.

CHAPTER 8

INTEGRATED PREVENTION AND CONTROL OF CARIES IN CHILDREN AND YOUNG ADULTS

For successful prevention and control of dental caries in children and young adults some basic principles must be adopted, based on the caries incidence of the targeted population.

CARIES INCIDENCE OF THE TARGETED POPULATION

High caries incidence and prevalence

The higher the risk of developing caries for most of the population, the greater the effect of one single preventive measure.

For example, 30 to 35 years ago, caries prevalence in Sweden was extremely high, and almost every child developed several new cavities every year, mainly because of very poor oral hygiene. Regular toothbrushing was not an established habit, and there was no effective fluoride toothpaste. Under the prevailing conditions, well-organized, school-based programs in which a fluoride mouthrinse (0.2% sodium fluoride solutions) was administered once every 1 or 2 weeks resulted in caries reductions of 30% to 50% (Torell and Ericsson, 1965; Forsman, 1965); these results

were comparable to the effects of fluoridated drinking water in other industrialized countries (the United States and the United Kingdom) with high caries prevalence at the time. In countries or districts with high caries prevalence and poor oral hygiene, the introduction of a single caries-preventive measure for all children, such as fluoridated drinking water, school-based fluoride mouthrinsing, or daily brushing with fluoride toothpaste, would still result in very significant caries reduction.

Low-to-moderate caries incidence

However, in populations with low or moderate caries incidence, well-established self-care habits, and well-organized oral health care, a single preventive measure administered to all subjects in the population, irrespective of predicted risk, will not be cost effective. In such populations, individual risk prediction and needs-related combinations of preventive measures are necessary. To ensure a high sensitivity of risk prediction, several etiologic and modifying risk factors have to be combined.

This is exemplified by the following: The Vipeholm study 45 years ago confirmed that pro-

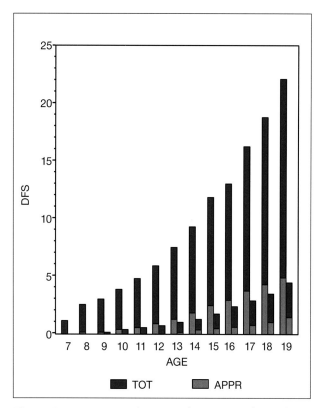

Fig 110 Caries prevalence in the county of Värmland, Sweden, in 1979 and 1996. (DFS) Decayed or filled surfaces; (TOT) total; (APPR) approximally.

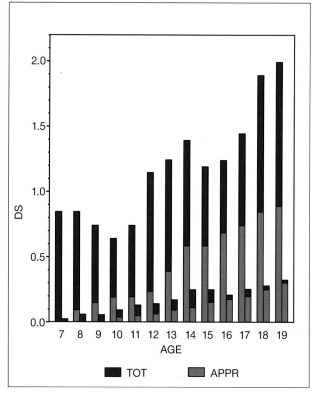

Fig 111 Caries incidence in the county of Värmland, Sweden, in 1979 and 1996. (DS) Decayed surface; (TOT) total; (APPR) approximally.

longed sugar clearance time is an external modifying risk factor for caries development in mentally handicapped people with heavy plaque accumulation, in the absence of oral hygiene or fluoride (Gustafsson et al, 1954). However, over the past two decades we have repeatedly failed to find any correlation between the intake of sugar products and caries prevalence in Sweden, because caries prevalence and caries incidence have declined dramatically as a result of integration of caries-preventive measures by self-care, support-

ed by needs-related professional treatment (Axelsson et al, 1993a).

Particularly successful has been the integration of a self-care program of excellent plaque control and the use of fluoride toothpaste, with professional mechanical toothcleaning and fluoride varnish at needs-related intervals. These results have been achieved despite the fact that the daily intake of sugar-containing products has remained unaltered over the last 40 years (about 120 g per individual each day) and that the percentage of sticky sugar products, such as sweets and cakes, has increased. In a totally integrated caries-preventive program, however, external modifying risk factors, such as high frequency of sugar intake, should also be addressed.

In the late 1970s, school-based fluoride mouthrinse programs once every 1 or 2 weeks were still recommended by the Swedish Board of Health and Welfare. However, in our population with high standards of oral hygiene, regular use of fluoride toothpaste, and low caries incidence, the supplementary cariostatic effect of the school programs was questionable. Therefore, from 1977 to 1980, a 3-year double-blind study was conducted to evaluate the supplementary effect of fluoride rinsing on caries incidence in 12- to 15-year-old subjects using fluoride toothpaste twice a day. There was no difference in results between weekly rinsing with 0.05% sodium fluoride solution and rinsing with distilled water (Axelsson et al, 1987a). The school-based mouthrinsing programs were consequently withdrawn, without detriment to caries prevalence (Fig 110) or incidence (Fig 111). Integrated, needs-related caries-preventive programs in County of Värmland, Sweden, have continued to achieve significant caries reductions of 70% to 90%.

INTEGRATED CARIES PREVENTION BASED ON PREDICTED RISK

The risk for caries development varies significantly for different age groups, individuals, teeth, and surfaces. Caries-preventive measures must be integrated and based on predicted risk from age groups down to the individual tooth surfaces. In other words, a medium-sized suit does not fit all the men in the world; it would be a reasonable fit for, at most, 40%, but too small for 30% and too large for the remaining 30%.

Based on this philosophy and experience from continuously ongoing research evaluating

and reevaluating separate and integrated caries-preventive measures, as well as methods for prediction of caries risk, an integrated caries-preventive program for 0 to 19 year olds was introduced in the county of Värmland, Sweden, in 1979. The goals for the subjects following the program from birth to the age of 19 years are:

1. To have no approximal restorations.
2. To have no occlusal amalgam restorations.
3. To have no approximal loss of periodontal attachment.
4. To motivate and encourage individuals to assume responsibility for their own oral health.

It is hoped that these goals will be attained for 20-year-old participants by 1999. The effect of the program is evaluated once every year on almost 100% of all 3 to 19 year olds in a computer-aided epidemiologic program from 1979 (Axelsson et al, 1993a).

Key-risk age groups

Studies by Köhler et al (1978, 1982) showed that mothers with high salivary levels of mutans streptococci frequently transmit the organism to their babies as soon as the first primary teeth erupt, leading to increased development of caries. Another study has shown that 1-year-old babies with plaque and gingivitis develop several carious lesions during the following years, while babies with clean teeth and healthy gingiva, maintained by regular daily cleaning by their parents, remain caries-free (Wendt et al, 1994). It is also well known that, on average, particularly the permanent teeth erupt 6 to 12 months earlier in girls than in boys. In addition, good oral hygiene and dietary habits should be established as early as possible and introduction of poor oral health habits should be prevented.

On this basis, the high-priority key-risk age groups are expectant mothers and 1- to 2-year-old babies, starting with girls (Fig 112). To prevent

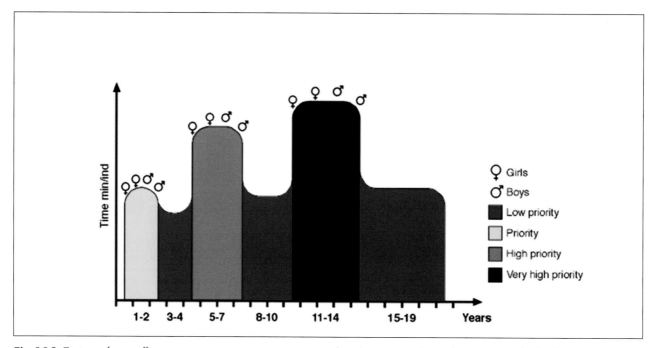

Fig 112 Timing of cost-effective caries-preventive programs, related to age and gender. Time min/ind = the needs-related mean time of preventive dentistry expressed in minutes/individual, related to age and gender.

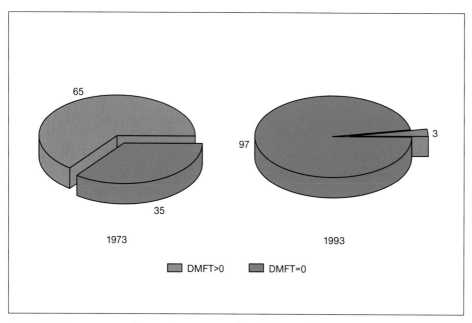

Fig 113 Percentage of caries-free 3-year-old children in the county of Värmland, Sweden, in 1979 and 1993 (left and right, respectively).

postnatal transmission of cariogenic bacteria and poor dietary habits from mother to child, expectant mothers at risk are offered a special preventive program at public dental health centers. Dental hygienists or preventive dentistry assistants provide prenatal counseling on an individual and group basis. At child welfare centers, dental hygienists or preventive dentistry assistants counsel parents on good oral hygiene and dietary habits for their children, and stress the importance of early introduction of fluoride toothpaste (in a pea-sized amount). As an effect of this program, the percentage of caries-free 3-year-old children increased from 35% in 1973 to 97% in 1993 (Fig 113).

Almost every carious lesion located in a fissure is initiated in the distal and central fossae of the permanent first and second molars during eruption (1.0 to 1.5 years), because plaque reaccumulation in erupting teeth is rapid and undisturbed, unlike that in fully erupted teeth in masticatory function, as shown previously in Fig 26. In addition, the enamel of erupting and newly erupted teeth is considerably more caries susceptible until so-called secondary maturation is complete. The caries-reducing effect of fluoride is also about 50% greater in erupting and newly erupted teeth than in teeth that have undergone secondary maturation (more than 2 years after eruption).

As a consequence, the next high-priority key-risk age groups are 5 to 7 year olds, during eruption of the first molars (the key-risk teeth), starting with girls (see Fig 112). Intensified mechanical plaque control twice a day with fluoride toothpaste should be performed by the children's parents, particularly on the erupting first molars. Home care should be supplemented at needs-related intervals by professional mechanical toothcleaning and application of fluoride varnish, and in the most caries-susceptible children, placement of glass-ionomer in the fissures.

The final, and highest priority key-risk age group is 11 to 14 year olds, from the age the second molars start to erupt in girls until they are fully erupted in boys (see Fig 112). In addition, the approximal surfaces of the newly erupted posterior teeth are most caries susceptible during this peri-od. These age groups have by far the highest number of intact, but at-risk, tooth surfaces. Therefore, integrated plaque control measures and use of fluoride agents should be intensified on the approximal surfaces of all the posterior teeth and the occlusal surfaces of the second molars.

Key-risk individuals

The role of etiologic factors and external and internal modifying factors related to caries risk, as well as the evaluation of risk profiles of the individual subject, has been discussed earlier in chapters 3 to 5.

In children, caries prevalence and caries incidence related to the age group and the combination of Plaque Formation Rate Index plus salivary mutans streptococci levels will give the highest sensitivity value for prediction of caries risk (see Fig 27). The percentage of selected key-risk individuals should also be related to age. In other words, the highest percentage of key-risk individuals should be selected in the 11 to 14 year olds and the lowest percentage in 3 to 4, 8 to 10, and 15 to 19 year olds (see Fig 112).

In children up to the age of 7 to 8 years, the parents have to assume responsibility for tooth-cleaning with fluoride toothpaste at least twice a day in key-risk individuals. From the age of 8 years, key-risk individuals should be motivated, educated, and trained to perform needs-related tooth-cleaning and to use fluoride toothpaste according to the principles applied in the Brazilian study described earlier (Axelsson et al, 1994). Fluoride chewing gum or fluoride lozenges should be used as a dessert directly after every meal.

In addition, key-risk individuals in all age groups require professional support: professional mechanical toothcleaning and fluoride varnish, chlorhexidine varnish, and glass-ionomer cement in the fissures of erupting molars, on the basis of individual need.

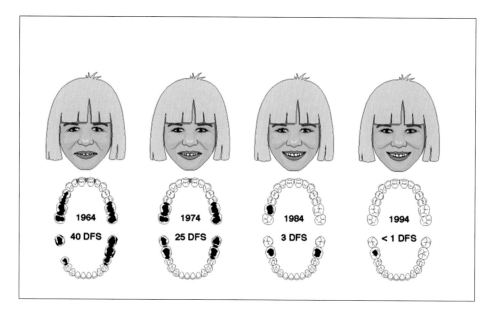

Fig 114 Caries prevalence among 12-year-old children in the county of Värmland, Sweden, at 10-year intervals, from 1964 to 1994. (DFS) Decayed or filled surface.

Key-risk teeth and surfaces

Figure 114 shows caries prevalence and the pattern of decayed or filled surfaces (DFSs) in 12-year-old children in the County of Värmland, Sweden, in 1964, 1974, 1984, and 1994. The molars are clearly the key-risk teeth. In a toothbrushing population, the key-risk surfaces are the fissures of the molars and the approximal surfaces, from the mesial surface of the second molars to the distal surface of the first premolars. Integration of mechanical plaque control by self-care and the use of fluoride toothpaste, supplemented at needs-related intervals by professional mechanical toothcleaning, fluoride varnish, and chlorhexidine varnish should therefore target these key-risk teeth and surfaces.

As shown in Fig 114, the mean caries prevalence in 1964 was about 40 DFS, generally involving all of the approximal and occlusal surfaces of the molars and premolars as well as some buccal and lingual surfaces. On average, one mandibular first molar was missing, extracted because of caries. During the following 10 years, the use of the toothbrush and fluoride toothpaste were introduced. As a result the number of DFSs

decreased to about 25. The reduction was mainly in caries on the approximal surfaces of the incisors and the buccal and lingual surfaces of the molars and premolars.

The separate effects of the toothbrush and fluoride toothpaste are difficult to estimate. In 1975 a needs-related plaque control program (both professional and home care), combined with fluoride toothpaste and fluoride varnish, was gradually introduced, targeting the key-risk surfaces of schoolchildren. The number of DFSs decreased to 3.0. The reduction occurred on the approximal surfaces of the molars and the premolars. The remaining caries, it is suggested, represents mainly overtreatment of first molar fissures.

A preventive program for the occlusal surfaces of the molars was initiated in 1984. In 1994, caries prevalence was less than 1.0 DFS. It is predicted that in 1999 the first group of 19 year olds who have followed this integrated preventive program from birth will have less than 1.0 approximal DFS (see Fig 110). The "filling" (F) component should account for less than 0.3 of this value, because approximal carious lesions without cavitation into the dentin can be treated noninvasively, without restoration.

Finally, it is important to emphasize the need for evaluation of new methods, as well as reevaluation of established methods, by clinical research in the actual population, before large-scale implementation, instead of direct extrapolation and implementation from animal and in vitro experiments. There are givens, but preventive measures should be tailored and integrated to reflect trends in the pattern of dental disease in a population.

CHAPTER 9

ORAL HEALTH GOALS

The World Health Organization's (WHO's) Oral Health Unit provides technical support for epidemiologic surveys and processes country data free of charge on request.

The information collected is stored in the Global Oral Data Bank (GODB) system in the catalog of United Nations data banks, whereby it is possible to follow worldwide trends. Every year since 1969, WHO has compiled a world map of caries prevalence in persons age 12 years. In 1969, the overall picture showed sharp contrasts: the number of decayed, missing, or filled teeth was very high, high, or at least moderate (from 2.7 to > 6.5) in the industrialized countries, whereas it was generally very low, low, and occasionally moderate in the developing countries, as discussed in chapter 1.

During the ensuing two decades, there has been a downward trend and sometimes a spectacular drop in the prevalence of caries in virtually all industrialized countries. In developing countries, the general trend has been an increase in caries prevalence, except where preventive programs have been established.

Any country undertaking an analysis of its oral health situation can compare the results with WHO's global goals: by the year 2000, no more than 3.0 decayed, missing, or filled teeth in children aged 12 years. By repeating the analysis at regular intervals (WHO recommends an evaluation every 5 years), it is possible to monitor the trend in caries prevalence, to estimate the need for care and prevention, and to adjust personnel training and services accordingly. The simplified oral health survey method developed by WHO is reliable, very inexpensive, can be used anywhere, and provides comparable data for both the wealthiest and the most impoverished countries.

Governments and communities should recognize the need to develop and maintain preventive programs for oral diseases—and communities will be responsible for these activities. All communities should be able to afford and manage basic, health-promoting oral care so that adult teeth will be retained throughout life. Early care should be available for oral cancer patients everywhere as well as for those suffering from other disfiguring, disabling oral diseases.

Changes in the training of oral health care personnel should ensure that dentists evolve into the role of oral physicians, providing guidance on lifestyle and hygiene, as part of maintaining health in general and oral health in particular. They should provide special care for the full range of oral problems.

Oral health for life should be approaching reality for all. To promote improved oral health worldwide, WHO's Oral Health Unit has drawn up international oral health goals for severity of oral disease involvement at various key ages—12 years, 35 to 44 years, and 65 years and older—by the year 2000:

1. The WHO databases for oral health will be further developed. Coordinated national database systems will be established. A WHO personal computer card for oral health recordings will be defined and produced.
2. Fifty percent of 5 to 6 year olds will be caries free.
3. Children will have no more than 3 decayed, missing, or filled teeth at 12 years.
4. Eighty-five percent of the population will have all their teeth left at 18 years.
5. A 50% reduction in edentulousness at ages 35 to 44 years will be achieved compared to the level in 1969.
6. A 25% reduction in levels of edentulousness at age 65 years and older will be achieved compared to the level in 1969.

In 1988, the first International Conference on Preventive Dentistry and Epidemiology was held in Karlstad, Sweden, in collaboration with WHO, Fédération Dentaire Internationale, and the Swedish Board of Health and Welfare. Among other topics discussed at the workshops were realistic goals by the year 2010 and 2025, to follow WHO's goals for the year 2000; what was known about already existing preventive measures; and the future potential of large-scale implementation of recent clinical research (Axelsson et al, 1988). The goals for the years 2010 and 2025 were proposed. The goals involve:

1. Creation of gradually more well-developed computerized analytic epidemiologic systems for quality control of oral as well as general health programs and cost effectiveness
2. Focusing on education of all the population in self-diagnosis and self-care, which is the most cost-effective oral health care

3. Prevention and control of caries as well as periodontitis development and progression in the vast majority of the adult population (secondary prevention) parallel with efficient primary prevention in children, resulting in about 90% caries-free young children

The following goals for the year 2010 should be achieved:

1. A complete electronic global, nation-based WHO database for oral health and a coordinated general health database will be established.
2. Ninety percent of 5 year olds will be caries free.
3. Children will have no more than 2 decayed, missing, or filled teeth at 12 years.
4. Seventy-five percent of 20 year olds will be caries inactive.
5. Seventy-five percent of 20 year olds will not develop destructive periodontal disease.
6. More than 75% of all children and young adults will have sufficient knowledge of etiology and prevention of oral diseases to motivate self-diagnosis and self-care.

The goals for the year 2025 should be:

1. A global electronic database for automatic oral and general health evaluation, including possibilities for health economy analysis, will be established.
2. Ninety percent of 5 year olds will be caries free.
3. Children will have no more than 1 decayed, missing, or filled tooth at 12 years.
4. Ninety percent of 20 year olds will be caries inactive.
5. Ninety percent of the whole population will not develop destructive periodontal diseases.
6. More than 75% of the total population will have sufficient knowledge of etiology and prevention of oral diseases to motivate self-diagnosis and self-care.

CHAPTER 10

THE INFLUENCE OF DENTAL INSURANCE SYSTEMS ON ORAL HEALTH STATUS

There is no doubt that different financing and insurance systems will significantly influence oral health status. Some of the different approaches to financing oral care are quality control guidelines, fixed fee agreements, capitation schemes, health maintenance organizations, rewarding increased preventive care, and public health funding. This chapter will discuss these approaches and propose an oral health insurance system based on the state of the art.

QUALITY CONTROL GUIDELINES

Using information about the duration of acceptable care products, quality control guidelines are being prepared, indicating the average number of years each type of care should last. If care procedures do not last the specified time, the clinician is then obliged to provide re-treatment free of charge. Such guidelines are intended to reduce unnecessary treatment that results in progressive destruction of tooth substance and higher costs for oral care.

FIXED FEES

In some countries, for most procedures, dentists may charge only fixed fees agreed between the health authorities and the professionals. These fees may be exceeded only for special treatment and after a review of the diagnosis and proposed procedure. In countries using this system, the costs of oral care are not rising, and costs are even decreasing in some countries.

However, dental insurance systems based on fixed fees for different specified treatment procedures, such as one anterior resin composite restoration versus complicated multisurface restorations, crowns, endodontic treatment, etc, are not a guarantee for improved oral health status among the population. For example, in Germany and Japan, the dental insurance systems are heavily concentrated on restorative dentistry, ie, so-called tertiary prevention. For items such as crowns and restorations, the dentists are relatively well reimbursed, but there is virtually no reimbursement for preventive dentistry according to the schedules issued by the national dental insurance scheme. As a consequence, dental practices concentrate on "drilling, filling, and billing" to survive.

This may explain why, in contrast to other industrialized countries, Germany and Japan maintain persistently high and close to high caries prevalence, respectively, in 12 year olds from 1969 to 1993 (see Figs 1 and 2 in chapter 1).

This is surprising, because both Germany and Japan have well-educated dentists, very high scientific standards in medicine, physics, chemistry, and economics, and a well-educated population with a high standard of living. On the other hand, it indicates the very powerful impact of the prevailing dental insurance system on the oral health status of the population.

CAPITATION SCHEMES

Capitation schemes pay the dentist a fixed sum for each person enrolled as a patient in the practice. For this fixed annual fee, a dentist contracts to maintain the oral health of all the enrolled patients. However, patients must undertake to attend for checkups on a regular basis, or they lose their rights and have to pay for treatment needed to restore their oral health. It seems likely that costs will be reduced by this type of program.

HEALTH MAINTENANCE ORGANIZATIONS

Health maintenance organizations contract with a group of oral care professionals to provide care to a group of communities or individuals, at agreed fees. Health maintenance organizations are usually organized and managed by companies that specialize in health insurance. This has proved an effective way to limit the costs of providing comprehensive oral care.

REWARDING INCREASED PREVENTIVE CARE

In some countries, projects to encourage preventive care give dental care managers a financial reward if disease levels do not increase in the patients in their catchment area.

PUBLIC HEALTH FUNDING

During the last decades, in most Scandinavian countries, oral health care programs for children and young adults, including school-based preventive programs, have been organized free of charge by the departments of health. This is one reason for the vast improvement in caries prevalence in Scandinavian children from 1969 to 1993. For example, in Sweden, the public dental health service has been granted a fixed annual allowance by the Department of Health to carry out needs-related dental care for all individuals up to 20 years of age. This has encouraged and motivated the public dental health service to focus on preventive dentistry and to delegate preventive treatment to dental hygienists and preventive dentistry assistants, to minimize costly restorative dentistry by dentists.

Particularly in the County of Värmland, Sweden, needs-related programs practiced by dental hygienists and preventive dentistry assistants have been successfully implemented under this capitation system. (See Figs 110, 111, and 114 in chapter 8.)

PROPOSED ORAL HEALTH INSURANCE SYSTEM

In 1973, a national dental insurance was introduced for all adults in Sweden, irrespective of whether they chose the Public Dental Health Service (40%) or private practice (60%). About 80% to 90% of the Swedish adult population visit dental clinics regularly for maintenance programs. To date, restorative dentistry, including crown and bridgework, has been based on an itemized fee schedule, but preventive dentistry and periodontal treatment have been based on an hourly fee, with different rates for specialist periodontists, general dental practitioners, dental hygienists, and preventive dental assistants respectively. The current insurance system was reviewed. A capitation system based on the individual's predicted risk combined with analytical epidemiology for quality control was introduced parallel to a modified version of the earlier system.

Oral health professionals must practice according to modern scientific principles and established, well-tried methods, ie, the state of the art. The causes of both dental caries and periodontal diseases are known, as are efficient preventive measures. High-quality oral health care must focus on prevention and control of dental caries and periodontal diseases and other oral diseases, ie, primary and secondary prevention. Existing treatment needs (tertiary prevention) must also be addressed.

In this context, it seems that all national dental health insurance schemes and finance systems should promote prevention and control of oral diseases, combined with analytic epidemiology for quality control, and cost-effectiveness analyses by the ministry of health, in accordance with the earlier described oral health goals for the years 2000, 2010, and 2025 (see chapter 9). In other words, the dental professional should expect to be well paid for successful prevention and control of oral diseases. An increasingly well-educated and well-motivated population will undoubtedly prefer an oral health care program giving priority to prevention and control of oral diseases to "extractions, drilling, filling, billing, and killing the pulp."

Ancient Chinese doctors were said to be very well paid as long as they were able to keep their patients healthy. If they failed, they received no reimbursement at all. The following proposal for an oral health insurance system is based on the state of the art.

The insurance would involve a capitation system based on the predicted risk, including needs-related primary, secondary and tertiary prevention. The individual annual fee would be combined with a negative fee based on the effect of the needs-related maintenance program on disease progression. For example, if the patient developed a new carious lesion, the patient's annual fee would be increased by 30 US $ and the dentist's reimbursement would be reduced by 30 US $. Likewise the annual fee would be increased by a certain amount for the patient and reduced by the same amount for the dentist, if the patient exhibited further loss of periodontal support.

For quality control of such an oral health insurance system, a computer-aided analytical oral epidemiologic system should be introduced. The dentist could present beautiful graphs in the waiting room to show the success of the practice in improving the oral health status and eliminating treatment need among the patients. It would significantly increase the dentist's reputation and good will. The patients would feel privileged to belong to the practice and pleased with the effects of their own efforts in self-care; they would be willing to pay a reasonable fee for the high quality of oral health care they were being offered.

Undoubtedly, no single preventive measure or combination of preventive measures would have such a significant impact on the improvement of oral health status as the aforementioned proposal:

1. Patients will be motivated to learn and improve self-diagnosis and self-care to improve their oral health status and prevent increased annual fees for oral health care.
2. Dentists will have a reasonable opportunity to practice state-of-the-art dentistry, and, as a consequence, their annual reimbursement will not be reduced.

CHAPTER 11

NEEDS-RELATED PREVENTIVE PROGRAMS

If all the countries with nonfluoridated water, high or very high caries prevalence and incidence, little or no daily toothcleaning, and no use of fluoride toothpaste were to introduce not only water fluoridation, but also daily supervised toothbrushing with a fluoride toothpaste in the schools, it would prove very cost effective for caries prevention and control. However, in industrialized countries with ample oral health personnel, oral health resources, relatively high standards of living and oral health, by far the most cost-effective strategy for improvement of oral health status is needs-related self-care based on self-diagnosis, supplemented with professional mechanical toothcleaning and topical application of fluoride agents at needs-related intervals. According to the state of the art, all new patients should be introduced to a needs-related preventive program in the following order.

SCREENING AND HISTORY TAKING

At the very first appointment, the goals are:

1. To obtain a brief overview of oral health status by screening diagnosis, supplemented with necessary radiographic examinations.
2. To gain an impression of the owner of the oral cavity by taking an oral and a general history.

It is important to remember that the diagnosis reveals only the present oral status, but the history discloses the reasons for that status. On the basis of the results of screening and history taking, appropriate detailed supplementary examinations and tests are selected.

EXAMINATIONS AND TESTS

The goals of supplementary examinations and tests are:

1. To obtain detailed information on oral health status.
2. To obtain detailed information on etiologic and modifying factors related to the patient's oral health status.

RISK CLASSIFICATION

Based on all data from the diagnosis and history taking, the patient is classified according to risk for dental caries and periodontal diseases: no risk (C0 and P0, respectively), low risk (C1 and P1), risk (C2 and P2), or high risk (C3 and P3). The individual risk profile is established as a tool for case presentation and communication with the patient (see chapter 5).

INITIAL INTENSIVE TREATMENT

The number of visits and materials and methods used is strictly related to patient's classification and predicted risk. The main goals of the initial intensive treatment are:

1. To establish needs-related self-care habits based on self-diagnosis and education.
2. To heal diseased periodontal tissues as soon as possible, resulting in a dramatic reduction in plaque formation rate.
3. To achieve arrest of carious lesions without cavitation.
4. To eliminate plaque-retentive factors, such as restoration overhangs, unpolished restorations, calculus, and rough root surfaces.

REEVALUATION

The goals of the reevaluation are:

1. To evaluate the results of the initial intensive treatment.
2. To assess patient compliance.
3. To evaluate supplementary need for regenerative therapy because of lost periodontal support and restorative treatment.
4. To determine the materials and methods needed for the maintenance period and the optimal recall intervals.

MAINTENANCE PERIOD

Intervals, materials, and methods of the maintenance program are strictly related to the patient's classification and predicted risk. The optimal goals of the maintenance program are:

1. To ensure that healthy individuals with no experience of oral diseases remain healthy (primary prevention).
2. To prevent recurrence of oral disease (secondary prevention) after initial successful symptomatic treatment (tertiary prevention); ie, to ensure no new caries lesions and no further loss of periodontal attachment.
3. To encourage continuous improvement in self-care habits to prolong the intervals and reduce the need for professional preventive measures.

RECALL EXAMINATION

Intervals, diagnosis, and supplementary history taking are strictly related to the patient's classification and predicted risk. The goals of the reexamination are:

1. To evaluate the effect of the maintenance program.
2. To prolong the intervals of the maintenance program and the recall reexaminations, provided that the patient's self-care has improved and there is no oral disease activity.
3. To evaluate whether new treatment needs have occurred.
4. To repeat an intensive treatment period and introduce a more comprehensive maintenance program if the previous program has proved unsuccessful.

IMPLEMENTATION

These principles for needs-related preventive programs are based on an ideal ratio of dental professionals, well-developed oral health care systems, high economic and educational standards among the population, and recent knowledge about diagnosis and preventive materials and methods. Local conditions may limit full implementation of this state-of-the-art program.

For example, in Sweden, almost all children and young adults and 80% to 90% of the adults are so-called recall patients; they receive some kind of regular maintenance program, but only a minority receive a strictly needs-related preventive program. In many other countries, however, maintenance programs are still nonexistent.

CHAPTER 12

DIAGNOSIS OF DENTAL CARIES

A carious lesion should be regarded as a symptom of the disease, dental caries. Table 4 shows the clinical diagnosis related to the type, localization, size and depth, and shape of the caries lesion. Carious lesions are diagnosed by the following methods, used separately or in combination:

1. Clinically, with visual inspection and probing
2. Radiographically, with a standardized bitewing view (specifically the approximal surfaces of the posterior teeth)
3. Radiographically, with digitized radiographs
4. Visually, with fiberoptic transillumination of the approximal surfaces of the anterior teeth

Figure 115 shows, in chronologic order, the development of coronal carious lesions: intact tooth (tooth 43), primary enamel caries (tooth 42), primary dentin caries with cavitation (tooth 41), secondary caries with cavitation (tooth 31), advanced secondary caries (tooth 32), and complete destruction of the crown (tooth 33).

Buccal and lingual enamel caries

Enamel caries on the buccal and lingual surfaces, as well as in the opening of the fissures, can easily be diagnosed by direct visual inspection after mechanical removal of plaque. When the caries attack rate is high (very active lesion because of very low pH), the surface of the enamel is rough, resembling unglazed china or chalk (Fig 116).

Under such conditions, most of the mineral loss is intraprismatic (Fig 117a). On the other hand, when the caries attack rate is slow, there is limited localized loss of interprismatic mineral. The outer and most caries-resistant part of the enamel forms a "micropore filter," through which minerals are released from deeper parts of the enamel and possibly the dentin (Fig 117b). Both of these types of carious lesions can be remineralized successfully by intensified plaque control and fluorides; in cross section, such remineralized lesions have different appearances (see Fig 100 in chapter 7). Figure 118 shows a cross section of an enamel caries lesion without cavitation, similar to Fig 117b. A close-up of the deeper part of the lesion shows that every separate enamel prism remains, but there is some mineral loss (Fig 119).

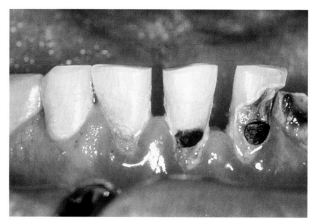

Fig 115 Development, in chronologic order, of coronal carious lesions: intact tooth (tooth 43), primary enamel caries (tooth 42), primary dentin caries with cavitation (tooth 41), secondary caries with cavitation (tooth 31), advanced secondary caries (tooth 32), and complete destruction of the crown (tooth 33). (Courtesy of D. Bratthall.)

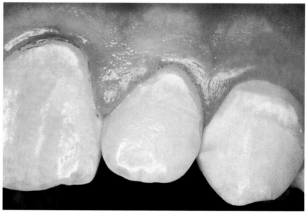

Fig 116 Active caries, resulting in rough enamel surface resembling unglazed china or chalk. (Courtesy of A. Thylstrup.)

Table 4 Diagnosis of clinical carious lesions related to type, localization, size and depth, and shape

Type	Localization		Size/depth	Shape
Primary caries	Crown	Occlusal surfaces Free smooth surfaces (buccal and lingual) Approximal surfaces Supragingival or subgingival	Enamel caries (incipient) Dentin caries (manifest)	"Smooth" surface "Rough" surface Cavitation Without cavitation Cavitation into the enamel Cavitation into the dentin Cavitation into the pulp
Secondary caries (recurrent)	Crown	Occlusal surfaces Free smooth surfaces (buccal and lingual) Approximal surfaces Supragingival or subgingival	Enamel caries (incipient) Dentin caries (manifest)	"Smooth" surface "Rough" surface Cavitation Without cavitation Cavitation into the enamel Cavitation into the dentin Cavitation into the pulp
Primary caries	Root	Buccal, lingual, mesial, distal Supragingival or subgingival	Cementum caries (surface or incipient) Dentin caries (manifest)	Soft surface (active lesion) Arrested surface Without cavitation Cavitation
Secondary caries (recurrent)	Root	Buccal, lingual, mesial, distal Supragingival or subgingival	Cementum caries (surface or incipient) Dentin caries (manifest)	Soft surface (active lesion) Arrested surface Without cavitation Cavitation

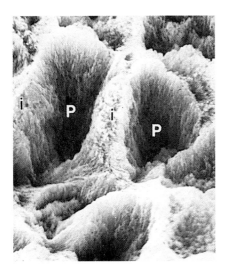

Fig 117a Intraprismatic mineral loss resulting from a rapid caries attack rate (very low pH). Observe that most demineralization is in the center of the individual enamel prisms (P). (Courtesy of Karger.)

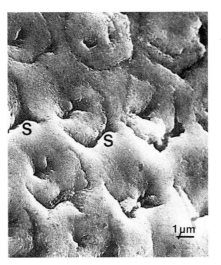

Fig 117b Limited localized loss of interprismatic mineral resulting from a slow caries attack rate with small interprismatic spaces (S). (Courtesy of Karger.)

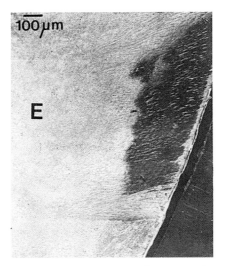

Fig 118 Cross section of a carious lesion in enamel (E) without cavitation. (Courtesy of Karger.)

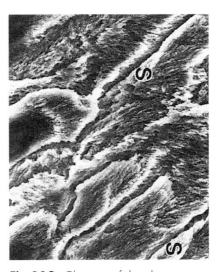

Fig 119 Closeup of the deeper part of the lesion shown in Fig 118. Every separate enamel prism remains, but there is some mineral loss from every enamel prism (P) and small interprismatic spaces (S) .

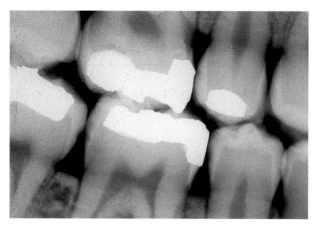

Fig 120 Radiolucent carious lesions in enamel on the distal surface of tooth 46 and the mesial surface of tooth 47. (Courtesy of J. Bille and A. Thylstrup.)

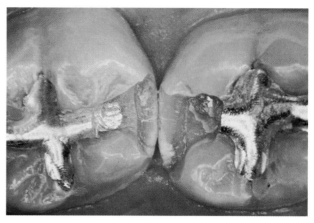

Fig 121 Cavity preparations to the depths of the lesions, as indicated on the radiograph, revealing that these are enamel lesions without cavitation, localized on the distolingual surface of tooth 46 and the mesiolingual surface of tooth 47. Note the close relationship among the localization of the lesions, the inflamed gingival margin, and the supragingival and subgingival plaque (the etiologic factor). (Courtesy of J. Bille and A. Thylstrup.)

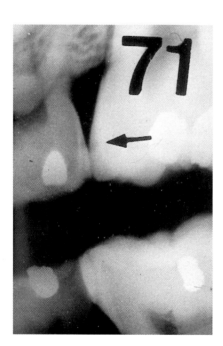

Fig 122a Enamel lesion (arrow) on the mesial surface of the first molar, adjacent to the primary second molar.

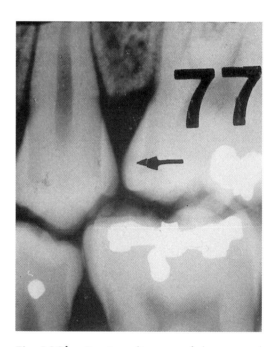

Fig 122b Remineralization of the enamel (arrow) on the first molar shown in Fig 122a. Remineralization occurred between exfoliation of the primary second molar and eruption of the second premolar.

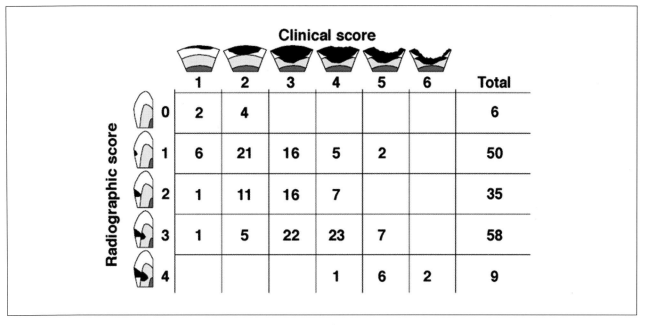

Fig 123 Comparison of radiographic and clinical scoring of approximal carious lesions. Radiographic scoring (Möller and Poulsen, 1973): (0) no radiographic changes in enamel; (1) radiographic changes in enamel; (2) radiolucent lesion that has reached the dentinoenamel junction; (3) radiolucent lesion penetrating approximately halfway through dentin; (4) radiolucent lesion close to the pulp. Clinical scoring: (1, 2) progressive changes in enamel; (3) changes in dentin without cavitation in the enamel; (4, 5) changes in dentin and progressive cavitation in the enamel, ie, still no bacterial invasion of the dentinal tubules and no indication for invasive tooth preparation; (6) cavitation involving dentin—possible indication for tooth preparation and restoration. (Modified from Bille and Thylstrup, 1982.)

Approximal enamel caries

The sum of the loss of minerals from every enamel prism is seen on bitewing radiographs as a radiolucent enamel carious lesion (Fig 120). Cavity preparation from the occlusal surfaces to the depth of the lesions, as seen on the radiograph, disclosed that these were enamel lesions without cavitation, localized on the distolingual surface of tooth 46 and mesiolingual surface of tooth 47 (Fig 121). Note the close relationship among the localization of the lesions, the inflamed gingival margin, and the supragingival and subgingival plaque—the etiologic factor. Arrest of such carious lesions in enamel can be achieved by use of a fluoridated wooden toothpick twice a day from a lingual direction, supplemented at needs-related intervals by professional mechanical toothcleaning (PMTC) with reciprocating pointed triangular tips and application of fluoride varnish.

Enamel carious lesions on the mesial surfaces of the first molars frequently remineralize over the short period (about 2 months) between exfoliation of the primary second molars and eruption of the second premolars (Figs 122a and 122b).

Approximal dentin caries

In a study by Bille and Thylstrup (1982), 8 to 15 year olds were examined clinically and radiographically. Approximal carious lesions were scored radiographically according to the system proposed by Möller and Poulsen (1973) (Fig 123).

During cavity preparation, the drilling procedure was discontinued when the full extent of the lesion could be seen on the base of the approximal box, cervical to the interproximal contact area. With the aid of an intraoral mirror and a

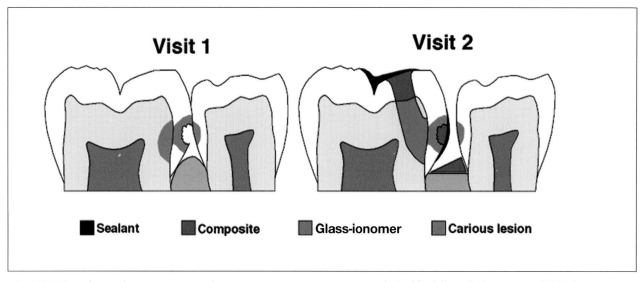

Fig 124 Partial tunnel preparation and atraumatic restorative treatment (Modified from S. Bjarnason, 1996.)

probe in normal clinical lighting, clinical tissue changes were recorded according to the six-point scoring system shown in Fig 123.

The relationship between radiographic and clinical scores is shown as a cross-tabulation in Fig 123. Although 58 of the 158 lesions showed radiolucencies penetrating approximately halfway through the dentin (radiographic score 3), none of these exhibited clinical cavitation into the dentin (clinical score 6). Only two of nine lesions with a radiographic score of 4 had a clinical score of 6 (Bille and Thylstrup, 1982).

Other studies have shown similar results (Mejàre and Malmgren, 1986; Pitts and Rimmer, 1992). For ethical reasons, Pitts and Rimmer (1992) used elastic orthodontic rubber bands to achieve temporary separation and thereby ensure accessibility for visible and clinical examination of radiographically diagnosed approximal carious lesions.

These studies confirm the importance of supplementing radiographic examination of approximal carious lesions with clinical inspection prior to treatment decisions.

Bjarnason (1996) used a technique similar to that used by Pitts and Rimmer (1992) for temporary separation, not only for clinical inspection

but also for minimally invasive operative intervention. A restorative technique that combined an external approximal composite restoration placed under rubber dam and so-called partial tunneling was used (Fig 124).

However, for lesions involving the dentin, but without cavitation, the approach should be, "prevention instead of extension," or "prevention before extension," that is, noninvasive (Figs 125 and 126). At the first visit, approximal surfaces with radiographically diagnosed lesions are cleaned professionally (PMTC), and painted with chlorhexidine-thymol varnish (Cervitec) for slow-release chemical plaque control.

To achieve temporary separation, an orthodontic elastic band is placed for about 5 days, in accordance with the technique described by Bjarnason (1996). At the second visit, after PMTC, approximal lesions showing no cavitation on direct clinical inspection are coated with chlorhexidine and fluoride varnish (Cervitec plus Fluor Protector), to remineralize and "seal" the outer "micropore" surface of the lesions (Fig 125).

If a limited cavity is diagnosed, it is mechanically cleaned with a small, ball-shaped finishing bur and filled with light-cured glass-ionomer cement, under the pressure of a translucent matrix

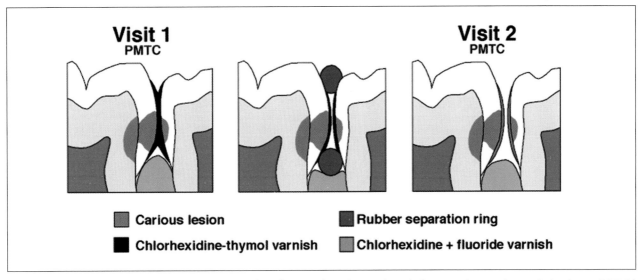

Fig 125 Prevention instead of extension. (PMTC) Professional mechanical toothcleaning. (According to P. Axelsson, 1995.)

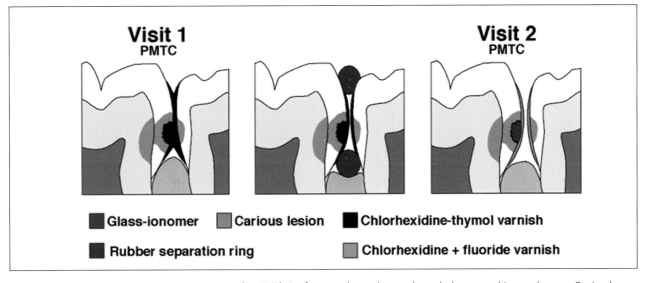

Fig 126 Atraumatic restorative treatment. (PMTC) Professional mechanical toothcleaning. (According to P. Axelsson, 1995.)

band. After an extrathin tungsten-coated recipro-cating tip is used for finishing (see Figs 67, 68, and 71 in chapter 6), the approximal surfaces are coat-ed with chlorhexidine and fluoride varnish, to seal the surface of incipient caries around the cavity margins (see Fig 126).

Fissure caries

Diagnosis of fissure caries, clinically (by probing), or radiographically, is a delicate problem because of the complicated three-dimensional form of the fissure system in which there is a great range of individual variations. Most molar fissures, in cross

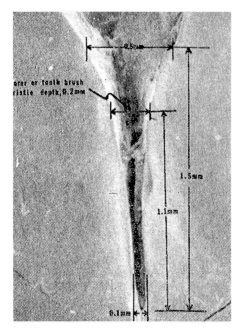

Fig 127 Cross section of a molar fissure.

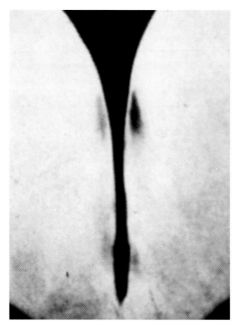

Fig 128 Atypical fissure with a narrow opening and a bulbous widening at the base. This type of fissure should be considered an at-risk fissure.

section, have a relatively wide opening, which narrows to a 0.1-mm-wide cleft approximately 1.0 mm deep—almost to the dentinoenamel junction (Fig 127). The carious lesion usually starts as an enamel lesion on both sides of the entrance of the fissure, which is visible and accessible to a probe. However, some atypical fissures (fewer than 10%), which have a narrow opening and a bulbous widening at the base, should be regarded as at-risk fissures, because a lesion can start at the base, as well as at the entrance, of the fissure (Fig 128). Fortunately, from a diagnostic point of view, there is a strong correlation between steep cuspal inclination and such "sticky" risk fissures.

In a study by Lussi (1991), experienced dentists recorded the status of the fissure systems of third molars and suggested appropriate management options. Subsequently, the teeth were extracted, histologically prepared, and examined. The results showed no difference in diagnostic accuracy between probing and visual inspection alone. The percentage of correctly diagnosed

teeth was only approximately 40%. It was concluded that probing does not improve the validity of the diagnoses of fissure caries compared to that of visual inspection alone and that the pressure of a sharp explorer may fracture the surface of the enamel lesion (the micropore filter), with subsequent progression to cavitation.

Figure 129a shows a clinically visible lesion, and Fig 129b shows the corresponding preparation in cross section: Although histologically the lesion is seen to involve the dentin, cavitation has not progressed to penetration of the dentin. Thus, there is still no clear motivation for invasive therapy; rather, prevention should be favored instead of extension. The procedure of choice would be PMTC and the use of glass-ionomer cement as a slow-release topical fluoride agent.

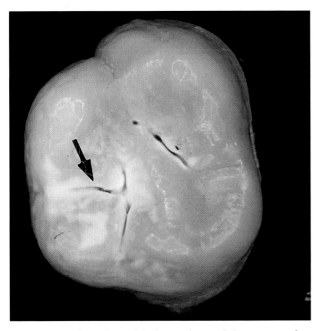

Fig 129a Clinically visible lesion (arrow). (Courtesy of A. Lussi.)

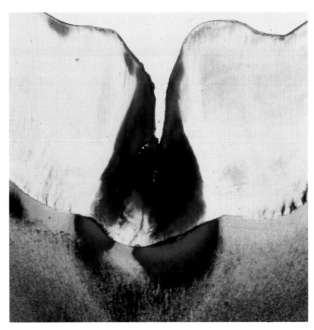

Fig 129b Cross section of the tooth preparation for the lesion shown in Fig 129a. Although the histologic view reveals that the lesion involves dentin, cavitation has not progressed to penetration of dentin. (Courtesy of A. Lussi.)

Root caries

According to Hix and O'Leary (1976), *root caries* is defined as "a cavitation or softened area in the root surface which might or might not involve adjacent enamel or existing restorations (primary and recurrent lesions)." Nyvad and Fejerskov (1986) introduced the definitions of *active* and *inactive* root caries. According to Table 4, root caries is classified as primary or secondary; cementum or dentin; active or inactive; and with or without cavitation. The lesions can also be classified according to the texture—soft, leathery, or hard—and the color—yellow, light brown, dark brown, or black. Active root carious lesions are light yellow with a soft or rough surface. Inactive lesions are dark brown with a leathery or rehardened surface.

When root surfaces are exposed to the oral environment as a result of recession of the marginal gingivae, the areas of potential plaque retention increase, particularly in the large interproximal areas and along the cementoenamel junctions (CEJs). The primary carious lesion of the root has a greater horizontal than vertical dimension because of greater supragingival plaque thickness immediately adjacent to the gingival margin. Initial active radicular carious lesions are soft on probing, have a leathery consistency, and normally are covered with plaque. The color is yellow or light brown. Because of extrinsic factors, such as staining from dietary components, smoking, and possibly from chromogenic bacteria present in the lesion, the color of the lesions will change to dark brown and black with longer exposure to the oral environment.

Studies by Nyvad and Fejerskov (1986) have shown that active root caries can successfully be converted to inactive caries as a response to improved oral hygiene and use of a fluoride toothpaste. Figures 130a to 130f illustrate various root carious lesions.

Figs 130a to 130f Various root carious lesions. (From N. Ravald, 1992. Reprinted with permission.)

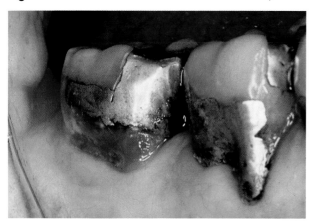

Fig 130a Active buccal lesion.

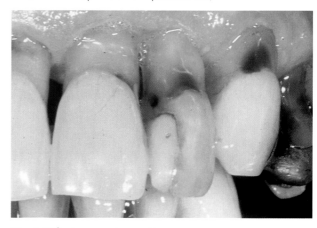

Fig 130b Inactive buccal lesions.

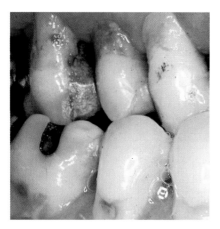

Fig 130c Active lesions covered with plaque.

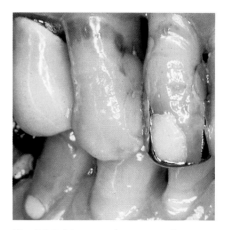

Fig 130d Inactive lesions and proper oral hygiene.

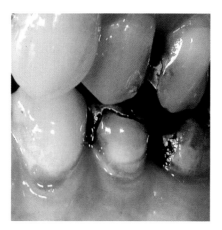

Fig 130e Active buccal lesion.

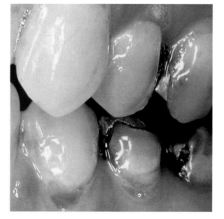

Fig 130f Same lesion as in Fig 130e, converted to an inactive state after 12 months of oral hygiene procedures and fluoride treatment.

Community Caries Index of Treatment Needs (CCITN) (Axelsson, 1988a)

For estimating caries treatment needs, a new index, analogous to the Community Periodontal Index of Treatment Needs (CPITN) has been designed (Table 5). The rationale is that estimation of treatment needs should encompass more than the restorative need: The emphasis should be on prevention. Carious lesions in enamel should be remineralized. The studies by Bille and Thylstrup (1982), Pitts and Rimmer (1992), and Lussi (1991), described earlier, showed that very few dentinal carious lesions on smooth surfaces or in fissures exhibited cavitation into the dentin. Therefore, most such lesions can be arrested. Nyvad and Fejerskov (1986) showed that, in response to improved oral hygiene, active root caries could also be successfully converted to inactive lesions. These findings further emphasize the importance of prevention instead of extension or at least prevention before extension, in contrast to the traditional concept of extension for prevention. Table 5 shows diagnosis and treatment needs at different levels.

The clinician must address the following questions in making a decision about invasive intervention:

1. How fast has the carious lesion progressed?
2. Why did the patient's self-care and my professional preventive measures fail to prevent development of the lesion?
3. How can we improve our combined preventive efforts to reverse, or at least arrest, the lesion?
4. How long should we wait to evaluate the results of our preventive efforts?

DIAGNOSIS OF PERIODONTAL DISEASES

Diagnosis of gingivitis

Gingivitis and periodontitis may be manifested clinically in various forms, which serve as the basis for their classification. Based on histologic and clinical criteria, gingivitis is classified in the following forms:

1. Initial gingivitis
2. Early gingivitis
3. Established (manifested) gingivitis
4. Acute necrotizing (ulcerative) gingivitis (AN[U]G)
5. Chronic necrotizing (ulcerative) gingivitis (CN[U]G)

The Gingival Index (GI), developed by Löe and Silness (1963), is most frequently used internationally for epidemiologic and experimental studies. The GI scores gingival inflammation from 0 to 3 on the facial, lingual, mesial, and distal surfaces of all teeth (Fig 131).

Table 5 Community Caries Index of Treatment Needs		
Score	Diagnosis	Treatment needs
0	Intact enamel	P?†
1	Primary enamel caries	P
2:1	Primary dentin caries; no C*	P
2:2	Recurrent (secondary) caries; no C	P
3:1	Primary dentin caries; with C	P + R?‡
3:2	Recurrent (secondary caries); with C	P + R
4:1	Primary (active) root caries; no C	P
4:2	Recurrent (active) root caries; no C	P
5:1	Primary root caries; with C	P + R?
5:2	Recurrent root caries; with C	P + R?

Modified from Axelsson (1988a).
*C = cavitation into dentin.
†P = prevention.
‡R = restoration.

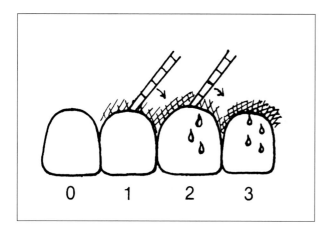

Fig 131 Silness and Löe Gingival Index (1963): (0) normal gingiva, no inflammation, no discoloration, and no bleeding; (1) mild inflammation, slight color change, mild alteration of gingival surface, and no bleeding; (2) moderate inflammation, erythema, swelling, and bleeding on probing or pressure; (3) severe inflammation, severe erythema and swelling, tendency to spontaneous hemorrhage, and some ulceration.

The Gingival Bleeding Index (GBI), developed by Ainamo and Bay (1975), is based on recordings of bleeding on probing from all four tooth surfaces of all teeth. Bleeding is recorded as present (+) or absent (–). A minus (–) is the equivalent of GI grades 0 and 1 and a plus (+) is equal to GI grades 2 and 3. The GBI is calculated as a percentage of affected sites (bleeding units). In adults, the GBI is very useful for experimental studies and individual practice application on a routine basis. In children, GI grades 2 and 3 are very seldom recorded, in spite of high prevalence of GI grade 1. Therefore, to avoid underestimation, for children the GBI should be modified to include GI grade 1 (Axelsson and Lindhe, 1974).

The patterns of dental plaque (Plaque Index), Plaque Formation Rate Index, and gingivitis (GI, GBI) are different from buccal to lingual and in maxillary and mandibular teeth. Therefore, six surfaces per tooth—mesiobuccal, buccal, distobuccal, mesiolingual, lingual, and distolingual—should be recorded in experimental studies, in analytical epidemiology, and in individual patient practice (Axelsson et al, 1990; Axelsson, 1991, 1994).

The Papilla Bleeding Index (PBI), by Saxer and Mühlemann (1975), is based on a 0 to 4 scale of bleeding 20 to 30 seconds after interproximal probing from a buccal direction in the second and fourth quadrants and a lingual direction in the first and third quadrants.

A simplified papilla bleeding index was developed by Gjermo and Flötra (1970), based on the presence (+) of papillary bleeding after inser-

tion of a triangular, pointed toothpick from the buccal direction. This index is very useful for screening procedures and oral hygiene education based on self-diagnosis by patients.

DIAGNOSIS OF PERIODONTITIS

Classification

Over the last 10 years, the following classification of marginal periodontitis has been used at the individual level. It takes into account the age of the patient, the pattern of periodontal attachment loss, and the incidence (progression rate) of periodontal disease:

1. Localized prepubertal periodontitis (LPP)
2. Generalized prepubertal periodontitis (GPP)
3. Localized juvenile periodontitis (LJP)
4. Generalized juvenile periodontitis (GJP)
5. Localized postjuvenile periodontitis (LPJP)
6. Generalized postjuvenile periodontitis (GPJP)
7. Adult rapidly progressive periodontitis (ARPP)
8. Adult (chronic) periodontitis (A[C]P)
9. Acute necrotizing (ulcerative) periodontitis (AN[U]P)
10. Chronic necrotizing (ulcerative) periodontitis (CN[U]P)

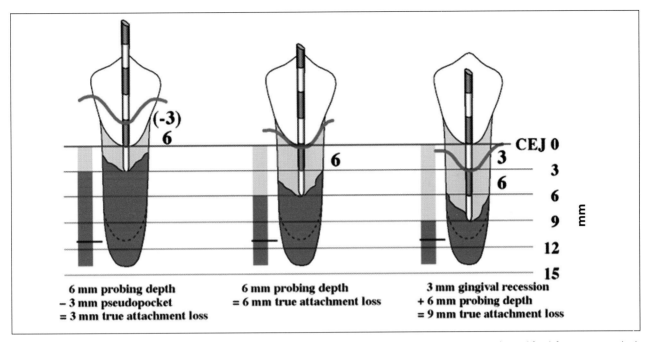

Fig 132 Relationship of probing depth to attachment loss. (CEJ) Cementoenamel junction. (Modified from Rateitschak with permission.)

Recent retrospective studies have shown that most patients with LJP had already lost periodontal support in the primary dentition (LPP) (Sjödin et al, 1989, 1993). Therefore, the first European Workshop on Periodontitis, Ittingen, Switzerland (Lang and Karring, 1994), recommended the following classification:

1. Early-onset periodontitis (EOP)
2. Necrotizing periodontitis (NP)
3. Adult periodontitis (AP)

Examination for periodontal disease must identify not only sites in the dentition with inflammatory changes but also the extent of tissue breakdown at these sites. The primary clinical symptoms of marginal periodontitis are loss of tooth-supporting tissues, attachment loss, and formation of suprabony and intrabony pockets. Therefore, careful measurement of probing depths and loss of attachment is essential.

Probing loss of attachment

The most important variable in the diagnosis of marginal periodontitis is clinical probing loss of periodontal attachment. In single-rooted teeth, loss of attachment occurs only vertically. In multirooted teeth, loss of attachment can also occur horizontally, indicating furcation involvement.

Vertical loss of attachment

Probing depth, unlike probing attachment level, does not disclose long-term failure or success of a maintenance program after periodontal therapy. This is exemplified in Fig 132; despite three different levels of periodontal attachment loss (3, 6, and 9 mm), the probing depth is 6 mm.

Vertical loss of attachment is the distance between the CEJ and the base of the pocket. It can be measured manually with a millimeter-graded probe. During measurement, use of an intraoral

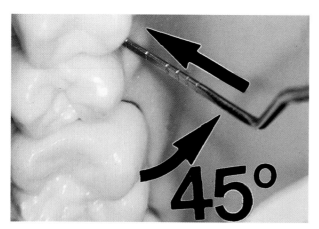
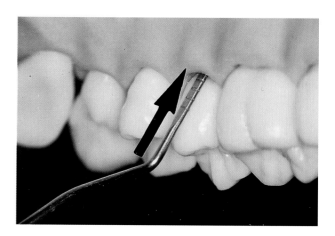

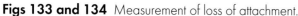

Figs 133 and 134 Measurement of loss of attachment.

mirror with fiberoptic illumination is recommended as an aid.

When the CEJ is located subgingivally, loss of attachment is measured as shown in Figs 133 and 134. The probe is held with a light pencil grasp, so that it can be moved and directed with minimal force. The end of the probe is then placed against the enamel surface coronal to the margin of the gingiva, so that the angle formed by the working end of the probe and the long axis of the tooth crown is approximately 45 degrees. With slightly decreased probe-crown angle, the distance between the free gingival margin and the CEJ is measured. The distance between the CEJ and the base of the pocket is measured as the loss of attachment level.

If the free gingival margin is apical to the CEJ or crown margin, attachment loss is measured directly from the visible CEJ to the bottom of the pocket.

The probe is used as parallel as possible to the long axis of the root. It is important that the point of the probe continuously follow the root surface, to prevent penetration of the pocket epithelium and connective tissue, resulting in underestimation of attachment loss.

The mesial surface is assessed mesiobuccally and mesiolingually, and the highest value is registered as representing mesial loss of attachment. The distal surface is measured only distobuccally.

The buccal and lingual surfaces are measured on the most prominent part of the root surfaces. In multirooted teeth, maxillary and mandibular molars, the highest buccal value is registered.

Electronically computerized periodontal probes have also been recently introduced (eg, the Florida-Probe and the Peri Probe). In one study, probing depths recorded by the Florida-Probe on teeth scheduled for extraction were compared with the true probing depth based on histologic evaluation after extraction. The results showed that, on average, the Florida-Probe underestimated probing depth by 0.5 mm (Hull et al, 1995).

Periodontal radiographs are useful for diagnosis of loss of periodontal support and quality control of a maintenance program: A standardized technique with long-cone and attached film holders should be used for periapical and vertical bitewing radiographs. However, studies by Goodson et al (1984) showed that advanced vertical probing attachment loss may occur interproximally in the molar area before loss of alveolar bone is discernible radiographically (Fig 135). This is due to the marked difference in degree of mineralization between spongiform and compact bone.

An alternative to conventional radiography is digital intraoral imaging, such as the Digora, Sedexi, and Sens-A-Ray systems.

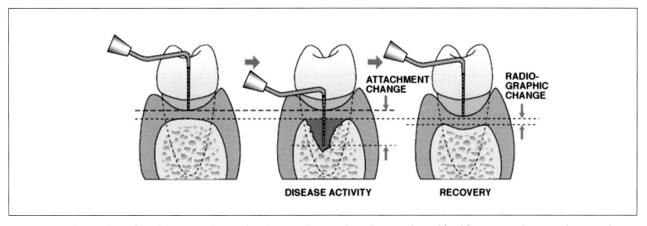

Fig 135 Relationship of probing attachment levels to radiographic change. (Modified from Goodson et al, 1984.)

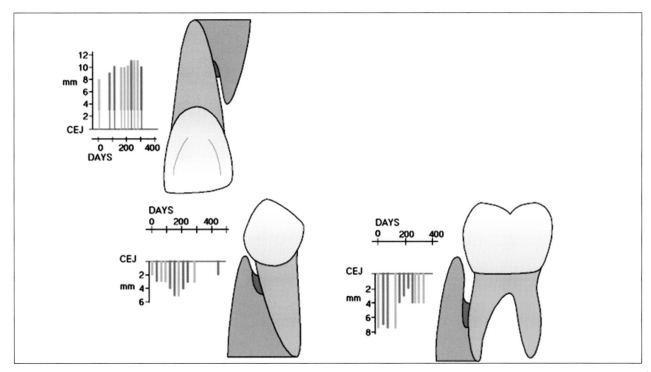

Fig 136 Progression and regression of attachment loss. The distance from the cementoenamel junction (CEJ) to the base of the pocket reveals the alterations in periodontal attachment during the period. (Modified from Goodson et al, 1982.)

As in caries and other infectious diseases, there may be exacerbations and resting periods (burnouts) in the incidence of periodontal diseases. Goodson et al (1982) measured probing attachment loss every month for 1 year in untreated subjects with existing periodontal pockets: among diagnosed sites, 83% did not change significantly, 6% exhibited significant further loss of attachment, and 11% exhibited less loss of attachment during the year. These results suggest that a dynamic condition of disease exacerbation and remission as well as periods of inactivity may be characteristic of periodontal disease.

137

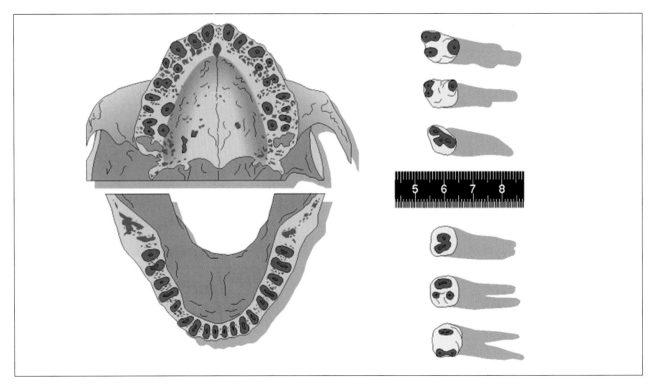

Fig 137 Cross sections of maxillary and mandibular teeth and variations in furcation topography on different teeth. (Modified from Rateitschak with permission.)

Figure 136 exemplifies the patterns of attachment level and probing depth in three different sites from the study. The distance from the CEJ to the base of the pocket shows the alterations in periodontal attachment loss during the period. According to this study, the potential to monitor changes in periodontal support at close intervals by complete-mouth radiographs is limited because of radiation exposure.

Other studies confirm that sites with destructive periodontal activity may show no further activity or subsequently may undergo one or more exacerbations. There may be relatively short periods in an individual's lifetime in which many sites undergo periodontal destruction, followed by prolonged periods of remission (Socransky et al, 1984).

Horizontal loss of attachment—furcation involvement

Progressive periodontal disease around two-rooted or multirooted teeth destroys the supporting structures of the furcation area. Treatment is often complicated. Therefore, the precise identification of the presence and extent of periodontal tissue breakdown within the furcation area of each multirooted tooth is of importance for proper diagnosis and treatment planning.

Three degrees of furcation involvement may be classified:

1. Degree I: Horizontal loss of supporting tissues not exceeding one third of the width of the tooth
2. Degree II: Horizontal loss of supporting tissues exceeding one third of the width of the tooth but not encompassing the total width of the furcation area
3. Degree III: Horizontal through-and-through destruction of the supporting tissues in the furcation

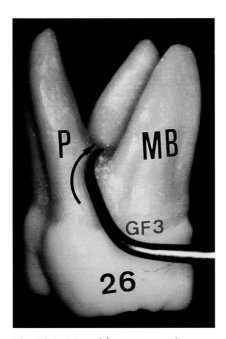

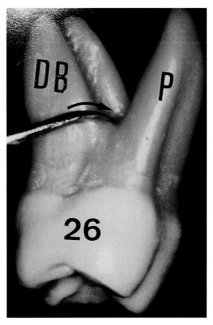

Fig 138 Mesial furcation involvement of the maxillary molar. This must be diagnosed in a mesiolingual-apical direction. (MB) mesiobuccal root; (P) palatinal root.

Fig 139 Distal furcation involvement of the maxillary molar. This must be diagnosed in a distobuccal-apical direction. (DB) distobuccal root; (P) palatinal root.

For accurate diagnosis, a slim, curved instrument is necessary. A slim double-ended curette, such as the Goldman-Fox No. 3, is appropriate. Special diagnostic probes for assessing furcation involvement are also available, eg, the flexible disposable tip of the TPS-probe and the Furcation Probe (LM). Figure 137 shows cross-sections of maxillary and mandibular teeth and variations in furcation topography on different teeth.

Mesial furcation involvements of the maxillary molars have to be diagnosed in a mesiolingual-apical direction (Fig 138) and, on the distal aspect, in a distobuccal-apical direction (Fig 139). Eccentric radiographs should also be used to detect furcation involvement. The levels of the entrance of the furcation area should be compared with the most coronal margin of the alveolar bone. Thereafter, the diagnosis is verified by probing.

Community Periodontal Index of Treatment Needs (CPITN)

The CPITN was developed jointly by the Fédération Dentaire Internationale (FDI) and the World Health Organization (WHO) in 1977 (Ainamo et al, 1982). The CPITN is now a recognized index to indicate levels of periodontal conditions in populations for which specific interventions might be considered.

The major features of the CPITN method include (1) use of the specially designed periodontal probe; (2) division of the dentition into sextants; and (3) assignment of scores for all teeth or index teeth in each sextant (Fig 140). Only the highest score for each sextant is recorded.

The code numbers recorded indicate the following types of periodontal treatment needs:

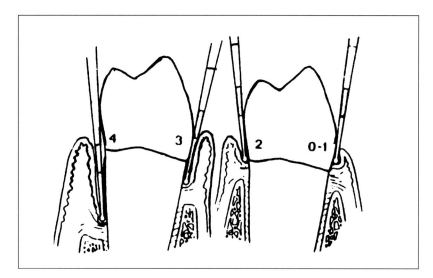

Fig 140 Community Periodontal Index of Treatment Needs: (0) healthy periodontal tissues; (1) bleeding after gentle probing; (2) supragingival or subgingival calculus or defective margin of restoration or crown; (3) 4- or 5-mm pathologic pocket; (4) 6-mm or deeper pathologic pocket. The code X is used when only one tooth or no teeth are present in a sextant. (Third molars are excluded unless they function in place of second molars.) (From Ainamo et al, 1982. Reprinted with permission.)

1. Code 0: There is no need for periodontal treatment.
2. Code 1: Oral hygiene instruction is required.
3. Codes 2 and 3: Scaling and root planing are required in addition to oral hygiene instruction. Scaling and root planing are also supplemented with elimination of plaque-retentive margins of restorations and crowns.
4. Code 4: Complex treatment is required in addition to scaling and root planing and oral hygiene instruction.

It has, however, been shown that, in individual subjects as well as in populations, "true" periodontal treatment needs are considerably overestimated when CPITN is used at the sextant level rather than the surface level (Axelsson et al, 1990; Axelsson, 1998). At the surface level, the CPITN is very useful for estimation of treatment needs in the individual patient.

Active lesions: Bleeding on probing and periodontal probing temperature

The classic clinical symptoms of a diseased periodontal pocket and active lesion are bleeding on probing, purulent exudate, and subgingival plaque biofilms. Other indications for active lesions are destruction of the most coronal level of the alveolar bone or the alveolus and the presence of subgingival microflora associated with progressive periodontitis: *Actinobacillus actinomycetemcomitans, Porphyromonas gingivalis, Prevotella intermedia, Bacteroides forsythes*, and *Treponemia denticola*.

The five classic signs of tissue inflammation are *rubor* (redness), *calor* (heat), *tumor* (swelling), *dolor* (pain), and *functio laesa* (loss of function). Redness and heat are related to vascular changes. The optimal temperature for regeneration of human pathogenic bacteria is 37°C, normal body temperature. A rise in temperature (fever), the nonspecific response to local and general infection, generally retards the bacterial regeneration rate. This was the basis of diagnosis of diseased periodontal pockets with a digitalized micro-thermometer with a flat, thin periodontal probe (Axelsson, 1982).

Recently, commercial thermal probes have been developed to assess subgingival temperature (Perio Temp system and Thermocoax TKA 05/10, Philips). These devices are about the size and shape of a periodontal probe and use a small thermistor bead to determine temperature. The probe tip is housed in a casing with low thermal conductivity so that the probe itself does not alter the ambient temperature. The probe is sensitive to 0.1°C and records the temperature rapidly so that the entire mouth (six sites per tooth, 168 sites for 28 teeth) can be evaluated quickly. The devices are linked to a computer.

In recent studies in which these devices have been used, the mean site temperature in active sites was significantly (about 1°C) higher than in inactive sites ($P \leq 0.001$) (Lindskog et al, 1994). The sensitivity for prediction of periodontal progression in one study was 85%, and the positive and negative predictive values were 87% and 53%, respectively (Buchmann et al, 1994). The findings from these studies are in accordance with existing knowledge of temperature increase in inflamed tissues and might improve the diagnostic potential for disclosing active sites at relative periodontal risk for further attachment loss.

In contrast, the commonly used periodontal diagnosis, bleeding on probing, is low in sensitivity, but relatively high in specificity (Lang et al, 1990). In other words, many pockets that bleed on probing are false diseased pockets, but a high percentage of pockets that do not bleed on probing are healthy.

ANALYTICAL EPIDEMIOLOGY FOR QUALITY CONTROL

Purposes

A great deal of time, effort, and money are spent on oral health care each year, so it is reasonable that the government agency responsible for health care have an audit system, which regularly evaluates the total effect of the national oral care and dental insurance systems on the oral health status and treatment needs of the population. At the same time, it encourages and motivates dentists to continuously evaluate the efficiency of their own preventive program at surface, tooth,

and individual levels, as well as for their total patient population. Also, a national dental insurance scheme should promote preventive dentistry and analytical epidemiology for quality control.

According to the *Swedish Medical Terminology* (1975), the definition of *epidemiology* is "the medical science of the spread, etiology, and prevention of the epidemic (infectious) diseases." Because certain types of transmissible microorganisms that colonize the tooth surfaces are implicated in the etiology of both caries and periodontal diseases, these diseases are regarded as epidemic diseases.

As discussed in chapter 9, WHO, in collaboration with FDI, international dental associations, and ministries of health, has established goals for the level of oral health to be attained by the year 2000 for selected indicator age groups in children and adults. One goal recommends that computer-based epidemiologic systems be established to monitor whether these goals are being attained.

Very powerful personal computers are now available and portable computers are suitable for field surveys. Today, large volumes of epidemiologic data may be collected, and direct statistical evaluation and graphic presentation of the results are readily accomplished with computer processing.

Disease prevalence

In contrast to other medical disciplines, dentistry has well-established and measurable variables for evaluation of oral health. These variables should be stratified according to their importance. The main reasons for loss of teeth are dental caries and periodontal diseases. Variables associated with these conditions should be given priority in oral health epidemiology. The masticatory efficiency of the dentition and the condition of the oral mucosa should also be included.

Tooth loss

The final outcome of untreated caries and periodontal disease is total edentulousness. According to WHO's goals, edentulousness in 35 to 44 year olds and 65 year olds should be reduced from 1969 levels by 50% and 25%, respectively, by the year 2000.

In field surveys, retrospective determination of the reason for missing teeth is frequently difficult and uncertain. Information with respect to which teeth are most frequently missing and the reason for extraction is important for planning appropriate preventive measures. Important questions that arise are:

1. Why are the maxillary molars the teeth most frequently missing?
2. Why are maxillary premolars missing more frequently than mandibular premolars?
3. Why are the mandibular canines the most resistant of all the teeth?

Loss of occlusal contacts

Mastication is the primary function of the teeth. Masticatory efficiency, ie, chewing capacity, may be expressed in terms of the Eichner Index, based on the number of occlusal contacts in the molar and premolar areas (Eichner, 1955; Österberg and Landt, 1976.

Dental caries and periodontal diseases

There is a strong correlation between oral health status and the occurrence of dental caries and periodontal diseases. The prevalence of these diseases is therefore the most important dental health variable. Many parallels may be drawn between these two diseases.

The etiologies are known; in both diseases, pathogenic microorganisms that colonize the tooth surfaces are implicated.

Both diseases are site-related, ie, not evenly distributed among the teeth and tooth surfaces.

For example, the difference in prevalence of both caries and marginal periodontitis between the distal surfaces of the maxillary first molars and the mandibular canines is usually more significant than the difference in total prevalence between individuals: There are specific, highly susceptible, key-risk teeth and surfaces. If the standard of oral health is to be improved by preventive measures, such facts must be acknowledged and the mechanisms explained. The prevalence of both caries and periodontal disease should be presented at the individual level as well as at tooth and surface levels.

The prevalence of both diseases represents the end result of all incidences and does not progress linearly. In other words, prevalence represents the results of unpredictable site-specific exacerbations and periods of disease quiescence.

Caries. For many years, caries prevalence has been expressed in terms of decayed, missing, or filled teeth (DMFT) and decayed, missing, or filled tooth surfaces (DMFS). In retrospect, it is difficult to ascertain whether the teeth and surfaces were lost because of caries. Caries prevalence should therefore be based on DFT and DFS. During the last few years, caries prevalence has been separated into coronal caries and root caries. At least in longitudinal epidemiologic studies, the depth of the carious lesion is differentiated as enamel caries and dentinal caries. Cavitated versus non-cavitated lesions should also be considered (see Table 4).

Periodontal diseases. The prevalence of marginal periodontal diseases refers to vertical loss of periodontal attachment in all teeth; horizontal loss of attachment with furcation involvement may also occur in multirooted teeth.

Because marginal periodontal diseases are site related, measurement of loss of alveolar bone on radiographs is not an acceptable substitute for assessment of clinical loss of attachment on every tooth surface. Buccal and lingual destruction of alveolar bone cannot be diagnosed on radiographs. In fact, the correlation between approximal bone loss diagnosed from radiographs and clinical loss of attachment is very weak (see Fig 135). Therefore, most epidemiologic surveys and longitudinal clinical studies on marginal periodontal disease prevalence and incidence are based on clinical loss of attachment.

In most countries, the prevalence of apical periodontitis has not been determined because complete-mouth intraoral radiographs or orthopantomograms are required for diagnosis.

Endodontic treatment

Data on the prevalence of endodontic treatment should also be collected. In an adult population, the number of root fractures is strongly correlated with the number of endodontically treated teeth with posts. Most coronal fractures also occur in root-filled teeth.

Mucosal diseases

From the oral health aspect, diagnosis of and collection of data on diseases of the oral mucosa are very important. In many countries, the prevalence of serious diseases, such as precancerous and cancerous lesions and human immunodeficiency virus–associated lesions, is increasing.

Treatment needs

To plan and organize the resources necessary to meet the need for oral treatment, an estimate must be made of treatment needs, not only for marginal periodontal diseases but also for caries, apical periodontitis, malocclusion, oral mucosal diseases, and bone diseases. Some new indices for treatment needs (CCITN and APITN, according to Axelsson, 1988a and 1988b)have therefore been designed, analogous to the well-established CPITN (Ainamo et al, 1982).

Etiology

In addition to epidemiologic data on prevalence and treatment needs, epidemiologic studies should also include causal and modifying factors, in terms of the previous definition of epidemiology. This is also confirmed by the definition of *epidemiology* in *Encyclopedia Britannica* (1963):

The medical science concerned with the description of factors and conditions that are significantly associated with the occurrence of an infectious process, disease or abnormal physiological state in a human community with elucidation of the manner in which these factors and conditions operate in the causative complex.

Oral epidemiologic system

In 1987, a new computer-based oral epidemiologic system was designed:

1. To evaluate the level of oral health status.
2. To assess the effect of preventive oral health programs at surface, tooth, individual, clinical, county, country, and international levels.
3. To determine indirect etiology and modifying factors of oral diseases.

A specially designed computer program is used for collecting the data. Another program is used for statistical analysis (Axelsson et al, 1988 and 1990). Table 6 shows, in ranking order, the variables included in the new oral epidemiologic system.

Prior to the clinical examination, the participants answer a questionnaire about their oral hygiene habits, dietary and smoking habits, systemic diseases and use of medicines, socioeconomic background, knowledge of causes and prevention of oral diseases, etc. In addition, complete-mouth radiographs are taken. Depending on the answers to the questions and

Table 6 Variables included in a computer-based oral epidemiologic system

Code	Variable
1	ORAL EPIDEMIOLOGY
1:1	% edentulous
1:2	Number of teeth
1:3	Function of the teeth: Eichner's Index
2	PREVALENCE
2:1	Dental caries, DMFT, DFT, DMFS, DFS
2:2	Marginal periodontitis
2:2:1	Vertical loss of attachment (mm)
2:2:2	Horizontal loss of attachment
	Furcation involvement score 0–3
2:3	Apical periodontitis
2:4	Oral mucosal lesions and bone diseases
2:5	Malocclusion
3	TREATMENT NEEDS
3:1	Dental caries: Community Caries Index of Treatment Needs (CCITN) (According to Axelsson, 1988a)
3:2	Marginal periodontitis: Community Periodontal Index of Treatment Needs (CPITN)
3:3	Apical periodontitis: Apical Periodontal Index of Treatment Needs (APITN) (According to Axelsson, 1988b)
3:4	Oral mucosal and bone diseases
3:5	Malocclusion
4	ETIOLOGIC FACTORS
4:1	Nonspecific oral microflora: Plaque Index (PLI) and Plaque Formation Rate Index (PFRI —according to Axelsson, 1987, 1991)
4:2	Specific microflora
5	MODIFYING FACTORS
5:1	External modifying risk indicators and risk factors: Poor oral hygiene and dietary habits, smoking and snuffing habits (other unhealthy lifestyle habits), socioeconomic background (particularly low educational level), use of medicines, infectious and other acquired diseases, etc.
5:2	Internal modifying risk indicators and risk factors: Chronic diseases (diabetes mellitus, cardiovascular diseases, Sjögren's syndrome, etc), impaired host response (particularly reduced PMNL function), reduced salivary secretion rate, etc.

the results of the examinations, clinical diagnoses are made by the examiner, and the data are entered directly into the computer by the dental assistant.

This system was used successfully in two large-scale analytic epidemiological studies on randomized samples of 35, 50, 65, and 75 year olds in the county of Värmland in 1988 and 1998 and in a longitudinal study of 50 to 60 year olds from 1988 to 1998 (Axelsson et al, 1988, 1990, 1998a, 1999b; Paulander et al, 1999; Axelsson, 1998).

REFERENCES

Addy M, Moran J, Wade W (1994). Chemical plaque control in the prevention of gingivitis and periodontitis. In: Lang N, Karring T (eds). Proceedings of the 1st European Workshop on Periodontology. London: Quintessence, 244–257.

Adriaens PA, de Boever JA, Loesche WJ (1988a). Bacterial invasion in root cementum and radicular dentine of periodontally diseased teeth in humans: A reservoir of periodontopathic bacteria. J Periodontol 59:222–230.

Adriaens PA, Edwards CA, de Boever JA, Loesche WJ (1988b). Ultrastructural observations on bacterial invasion in cementum and radicular dentine of periodontally diseased human teeth. Periodontol 55:493–503.

Ah MKB, Johnson GK, Kaldahl WB, Patil KD, Kalkwarf KL (1994). The effect of smoking on the response to periodontal therapy. J Clin Periodontol 21:91–97.

Ainamo J, Bay I (1975). Problems and proposals for recording gingivitis and plaque. Int Dent J 25:229–235.

Ainamo J, Barmes D, Beagrie G, Cutress T, Martin J, Sardo-Infirri J (1982). Development of the WHO community periodontal index of treatment needs (CPITN). Int Dent J 32:281–293.

Alaluusua S, Asikainen S, Lai C (1991). Intrafamilial transmission of Actinobacillus actinomycetemcomitans. J Periodontol 62:207–210.

Axelsson P, Lindhe J (1974). The effect of a preventive program on dental plaque, gingivitis and caries in schoolchildren. Results after 1 and 2 years. J Clin Periodontol 1:126–138.

Axelsson P, Lindhe J, Wäseby J (1976). The effect of various plaque control measures on gingivitis and caries in schoolchildren. Community Dent Oral Epidemiol 4:232–239.

Axelsson P, Lindhe J (1977). The effect of a plaque control program on gingivitis and dental caries in schoolchildren. J Dent Res 6(special issue): 142–148.

Axelsson P, Lindhe J (1978). Effect of controlled oral hygiene procedures on caries and periodontal disease in adults. J Clin Periodontol 5:133–151.

Axelsson P (1981). Concept and practice of plaque control. Pediatr Dent 3:101–113.

Axelsson P, Lindhe J (1981a). Effect of oral hygiene and professional tooth-cleaning on gingivitis and dental caries. Community Dent Oral Epidemiol 6:251–255.

Axelsson P, Lindhe J (1981b). The significance of maintenance care in the treatment of periodontal disease. J Clin Periodontol 8:281–294.

Axelsson P, Lindhe J (1981c). Effect of controlled oral hygiene procedures on caries and periodontal disease in adults—Results after six years. J Clin Periodontol 8:239–248.

Axelsson P (1983). Plaque Formation Rate Index (PFRI). A pilot study (manuscript).

Axelsson P, Lindhe J (1987). Efficacy of mouthrinses in inhibiting dental plaque and gingivitis in man. J Clin Periodontol 14:205–212.

Axelsson P, Paulander J, Nordqvist K, Karlsson R (1987a). The effect of fluoride-containing dentifrice, rinsing and varnish on interproximal dental caries. A 3-year clinical trial. Comm Dent Oral Epidemiol 15:177–180.

Axelsson P, Kristoffersson K, Karlsson R, Bratthall D (1987b). A 30-month longitudinal study of the effects of some oral hygiene measures on *Streptococcus mutans* and approximal dental caries. J Dent Res 66:761–765.

Axelsson P (1987). Plaque Formation Rate Index (PFRI)—Indicator for prevention of caries, gingivitis, and periodontitis, frequency and pattern of needs-related oral hygiene [in Swedish]. Tandlakartidningen 79:7:387–391.

Axelsson P, Paulander J, Tollskog G (1988). A new computer-based oral epidemiology system. Presented at the 1st International Conference on Preventive Dentistry and Epidemiology, Karlstad, Sweden.

References

Axelsson P, Paulander J, Tollskog G (1990). A new computer-based oral epidemiology system. Presented at the 2nd International Conference on Preventive Dentistry and Epidemiology, Karlstad, Sweden.

Axelsson P (1991). A four-point scale for selection of caries risk patients, based on salivary *S. mutans* levels and plaque formation rate index. In: Risk Markers for Oral Diseases—Caries. Vol I. 158–170. Cambridge: Cambridge University Press.

Axelsson P, Lindhe J, Nyström B (1991). On the prevention of caries and periodontal disease. Results of a 15-year longitudinal study in adults. J Clin Periodontol 13:182–189.

Axelsson P (1993). New ideas and advancing technology in prevention and nonsurgical treatment of periodontal disease. Int Dent J 43:223–238.

Axelsson P, Paulander J, Svärdström G, Tollskog G, Nordensten S (1993a). Integrated caries prevention: The effect of a needs-related preventive program on dental caries in children, County of Värmland, Sweden—Results after 12 years. Caries Res 27 (Suppl 1): 83–94.

Axelsson P, Rolandsson M, Bjerner B (1993b). How Swedish dental hygienists apply their training program in the field. Comm Dent Oral Epidemiol 21:297–302.

Axelsson P (1994). Mechanical plaque control. In: Lang NP, Karring T (eds). Proceedings of the 1st European Workshop on Periodontology. Chicago: Quintessence.

Axelsson P, Paulander J (1994). The oral health status in 50- to 55-year-olds in the county of Värmland (manuscript).

Axelsson P, Buischi YAP, Barbosa MFZ, Karlsson R, Pradi MCB (1994). The effect of a new oral hygiene training program on approximal caries in 12–15-year-old Brazilian children: Results after 3 years. Adv Dent Res 8(2):278–284.

Axelsson P, Paulander J, Hontwedt M, Östlund L, Engström A (1997). The effect of F-chewing gum on salivary secretion rate, plaque (PI), plaque formation rate (PFRI), salivary mutans streptococci (MS) and oral mucosa in subjects with reduced salivary secretion rate—A 6-month longitudinal study [abstract]. Presented at the 5th World Congress on Preventive Dentistry, Cape Town, South Africa.

Axelsson P (1998). Needs-related plaque control measures based on risk prediction. In: Lang PN, Attström, Löe H (eds). Proceedings of the European Workshop on Mechanical Plaque Control. Chicago: Quintessence, 190–247.

Axelsson P, Paulander J, Lindhe J (1998). Relationship between smoking and dental status in 35-, 50-, 65-, and 75-year-old individuals. J Clin Periodontol 25:297–305.

Axelsson P, Struzycka I, Wojcieszek D, Wierzbicka M (1999a). Prediction of caries risk based on salivary mutans streptococci (MS) levels and plaque formation rate index (PFRI) (manuscript).

Axelsson P, Paulander J, Svärdström G, Kaijser H (1999b). The impact of epidemiological data on prevention of periodontal disease. J Parodontol Implantol Orale (in press).

Bass CC (1954). An effective method of personal oral hygiene. J La Med Soc 106:100–112.

Beck J, Garcia R, Heiss G et al. (1996). Periodontal disease and cardiovascular disease. J Periodontol 67(suppl):1123–1137.

Bellini HT, Arneberg P, von der Fehr FR (1981). Oral hygiene and caries. A review. Acta Odontol Scand 39:257–265.

Bergström J, Preberg H (1994). People at risk for periodontitis—Tobacco as a risk factor. J Periodontol 65:545–550.

Bille J, Thylstrup A (1982). Radiographic diagnosis and clinical tissue changes in relation to treatment of approximal carious lesions. Caries Res 16:1–6.

Bjarnason S (1996). Temporary tooth separation in the treatment of approximal carious lesions. Quintessence Int 27(4):249–251.

Black GV, McKay FS (1916). Mottled teeth: An endemic developmental imperfection of the enamel of the teeth, heretofore unknown in the literature in dentistry. Dent Cadmos 58:129–156.

Bouwsma O, Yost K, Baron H (1992). Comparison of a chlorhexidine rinse and a wooden interdental cleaner in reducing interdental gingivitis. Am J Dent 5:143–146.

Bowden G (1991). Which bacteria are carcinogenic in humans? In: Johnson N (ed). Risk Markers for Oral Diseases—Caries. Vol I. Cambridge: Cambridge Univ Press, 266–286.

Bratthall D (1991). The global epidemiology of mutans streptococci. In: Johnson NW (ed). Risk Markers for Oral Diseases—Caries. Vol I. Cambridge: Cambridge Univ Press, 287–312.

Bratthall D, Ericsson D (1994). Tests for assessment of caries risk. In: Thylstrup A, Fejerskov O (eds). Textbook of Clinical Cariology. Copenhagen: Munksgaard, 333–353.

Bratthall D, Hänsel-Petersson G, Sundberg H (1996). Reasons for the caries decline: What do the experts believe? Eur J Oral Sci 104:416–422.

Buchmann R, Heinecke A, Lange DE (1994). Subgingival temperature and bleeding on probing as periodontal risk factors [abstract]. Eurioperio 7, Paris, France.

Buischi YAP, Axelsson P, Zülske Barbosa M, Mayer M, Carmen M, de Oliviera L (1989). Salivary *S. mutans* and caries prevalence in Brazilian schoolchildren. Community Dent Oral Epidemiol 17:20–30.

Buonocore MG (1955). A simple method of increasing the adhesion of acrylic filling materials to enamel surfaces. J Dent Res 34:849–53.

Carvalho JC, Ekstrand KR, Thylstrup A (1989). Dental plaque and caries on occlusal surfaces of first permanent molar in relation to stage of eruption. J Dent Res 68:773–779.

Carvalho JC, Thylstrup A, Ekstrand KR (1992). Results after 3 years of non-operative occlusal caries treatment of erupting first permanent molars. Community Dent Oral Epidemiol 20:187–92.

Clarkson BH, Fejerskov O, Ekstrand J, Burt B (1996). Rational use of fluorides in caries control. In Fejerskov O, Ekstrand J, Burt B (eds). Fluoride in Dentistry. Copenhagen: Munksgaard.

Coldiron NB, Yukna RA, Weir J, Caudill RF (1990). A quantitative study of cementum removal with hand curettes. J Periodontol 6:293–299.

Corey LA, Nance WE, Hofstede P, Schenkein H (1993). Periodontal disease in a Virginia twin population. J Periodontol 64:1205–1208.

Cunea E, Axelsson P (1997). Plaque Formation Rate Index (PFRI) in 3- to 19-year-olds [in German]. Phillip J 7-8:237–239.

Dawes C, Jenkins GN, Tonge CH (1963). The nomenclature of the integuments of the enamel surface of teeth. Br Dent J 16:65–68.

Dean HT, Elvove E (1936). Some epidemiological aspects of chronic endemic dental fluorosis. Am J Public Health 26:567–575.

Dean HT, Jay P, Arnold FA Jr, Elvove E (1941). Domestic water and dental caries. II. A study of 2832 white children aged 12–14 years, of 8 suburban Chicago communities, including L acidophilus studies of 1761 children. Public Health Rep 56:761–792.

Dean HT (1942). The investigation of physiological effects by the epidemiological method. In: Moulton FR (ed). Fluorine and Dental Health. 23–31. Washington, DC: American Association for the Advancement of Science.

Dean HT, Arnold FA Jr, Elvove E (1942). Domestic water and dental caries. V. Additional studies of the relation of fluoride domestic waters to dental caries experience in 4425 white children aged 12–14 years of 13 cities in 4 states. Public Health Rep 57:1155–1179.

Duckworth RM, Knoop DTM, Stephen KW (1991). Effect of mouthrinsing after toothbrushing with a fluoride dentifrice in human salivary fluoride levels. Caries Res 25:287–291.

Duckworth RM, Jones Y, Nicholson J, Jacobson APM, Chestnut IG (1994). Studies on plaque fluoride after use of F-containing dentifrices. Adv Dent Res 8:202–207.

Ehnevid H, Jansson L, Lindskog S, Blomlöf L (1993a). Periodontal healing in relation to radiographic attachment and endodontic infection. J Periodontol 64:1199–1204.

Ehnevid H, Lindskog S, Jansson L, Blomlöf L (1993b). Tissue formation on cementum surfaces in vivo. Swed Dent J 17:1–8.

Ehnevid H, Jansson L, Lindskog S, Weintraub A, Blomlöf L (1995). Endodontic pathogens: Propagation of infection through patent dentinal tubules in traumatized monkey teeth. Endod Dent Traumatol 11:229–234.

Eichner K (1955). Prosthodontic need index because of lost teeth [in German]. Dtsch Zahnärztl Z 10:1831–1834.

Elworthy A, Edgar R, Moran J, Addy M, Movert R, Kelty E, Wade W (1995). A 6-month home-usage trial of 0.7% and 0.2% delmopinol mouthwashes. II. Effects on the plaque microflora. J Clin Periodontol 22:527–532.

Emilson CG (1994). Potential efficacy of chlorhexidine against mutans streptococci and human dental caries. J Dent Res 73:682–691.

Evans RW, Stam JW (1991). An epidemiologic estimate of the critical period during which human maxillary central incisors are most susceptible to fluorosis. J Public Health Dent 51:251–259.

Federation Dentaire Internationale. Review of methods of identification of high caries risk groups and individuals. Federation Dentaire Internationale Technical Report No 31. Int Dent J 1988;38: 177–189.

Federation Dentaire International. Basic Facts 1990: Dentistry around the world.

Fejerskov O, Clarkson BH (1996). Dynamics of caries lesion formation. In: Fejerskov O, Ekstrand J, Burt B (eds). Fluoride in Dentistry. Copenhagen: Munksgaard.

Fejerskov O, Baelum V, Richards A (1996). Dose-response and dental fluorosis. In: Fejerskov O, Ekstrand J, Burt B. Fluoride in Dentistry. Copenhagen: Munksgaard.

Forsman B (1965). Effect of mouthrinses with sodium fluoride at schools in Värmland, Sweden. Tandlakartidningen 57:705–709.

Gillespie GM, Roviralta G (1985). Salt fluoridation. Scientific Publication no. 501, Washington DC: Pan American Health Organization (WHO-AMRO).

Gjermo P (1986). Promotion of Self-Care in Oral Health. Oslo: Scandinavian Working Group for Preventive Dentistry, Dental Faculty,

References

Gjermo P, Flötra L (1970). The effect of different methods of interdental cleaning. J Periodontal Res 5:230–236.

Goodson JM, Tanner ACR, Haffajee AD, Sornberger GC, Socransky SS (1982). Patterns of progression and regression of advanced destructive periodontal disease. J Clin Periodontol 9:472–481.

Goodson JM, Tanner ACR, Haffajee AD, Sornberger GC, Socransky SS (1982). Patterns of progression and regression of advanced destructive periodontal disease. J Clin Periodontol 9:472–481.

Goodson JM, Haffajee AD, Socransky SS (1984). The relationship between attachment level loss and alveolar bone loss. J Clin Periodontol 11:348–359.

Grossi SG, Zambon JJ, Ho AW, Koch G, Dunford RG, Machtei EE, et al (1994). Assessment of risk for periodontal disease. I. Risk indicators of attachment loss. J Periodontol 65:260–267.

Gustafsson BE, Quensel CE, Lanke LS, Lundqvist C, Grahnén H, Bonow BE, Krasse B (1954). The Vipeholm dental caries study. The effect of different levels of carbohydrate intake on caries activity in 436 individuals observed for 5 years. Acta Odontol Scand 11:232.

Hänggi D, Ritz L, Rateitschak KH (1991). Perioplaner/periopolisher. Loss of mineralized tissue from the root surface. First clinical experience [in German]. Schweiz Monatsschr Zahnmed 101:1535–1541.

Hix J, O'Leary T (1976). The relationship between cemental caries, oral hygiene status and fermentable carbohydrate intake. J Periodontol 47:398–404.

Hodge HC (1950). The concentration of fluorides in the drinking water to give the point of minimum caries with maximum safety. J Am Dent Assoc 40:436–439.

Hull PS, Clerehugh V, Ghassemi-Aval A (1995). An assessment of the validity of a constant force electronic probe in measuring probing depths. J Periodontol 66:848–851.

Imfeld T (1978). In vivo assessment of plaque acid production. A long-term retrospective study. In: Guggenheim R (ed). Proceedings of the ERGOB Conference on Health and Sugar Substitutes. 218–223. Basel: Karger.

Jeffcoat MK, Bray KS, Ciancio SG, Dentino AR, Fine DH, Gordon JM, et al (1998). Adjunctive use of subgingival controlled-release chlorhexidine chip reduces probing depth and improves attachment level compared with scaling and root-planing alone. J Periodontol 69:989–997.

Johnson MF (1993). Comparative efficacy of NaF and SMFP dentifrices in caries prevention: A meta-analytic overview. Caries Res 27:328–336.

Kashani H, Birkhed D, Petersson LG (1998). Fluoride concentration in the approximal area after using toothpicks and other fluoride-containing products. Eur J Oral Sci 106:564.

Keyes PH (1960). The infectious and transmissible nature of experimental dental caries. Findings and implications. Arch Oral Biol 1:304.

Kieser JB (1994). Review of nonsurgical therapy. In: Lang NP, Karring T (eds). 1st European Workshop on Periodontology. Chicago: Quintessence.

Kjaerheim V (1995). Experiments with triclosan [thesis]. Oslo: University of Oslo.

Klavan B (1975). Clinical observations following root amputation in maxillar molar teeth. J Periodontol 46:1–5.

Klock B, Krasse B (1979). A comparison between different methods for prediction of caries activity. Scand J Dent Res 87:129–139.

Köhler B, Bratthall D (1978). Intrafamilial levels of *Streptococcus mutans* and some aspects of the bacterial transmission. Scand J Dent Res 86:35–42.

Köhler B, Andréen I, Jonsson B, Hultqvist E (1982). Effect of caries preventive measures on *Streptococcus mutans* and *lactobacilli* in selected mothers. Scand J Dent Res 90:102–108.

Köhler B, Bratthall D, Krasse B (1983). Preventive measures in mothers influence the establishment of *Streptococcus mutans* in their infants. Arch Oral Biol 28:225–231.

Kornman KS, Crane A, Wang H-Y, et al (1997). The interleukin-1 genotype as a severity factor in adult periodontal disease. J Clin Periodontol 24:72–77.

Kosikowski F (1970). Cheese and Fermented Milk Foods. Ann Arbor: Edwards Bros.

Kotsanos N, Darling AI (1991). Influence of posteruptive age of enamel on its susceptibility to artificial caries. Caries Res 25:241–250.

Kristoffersson K, Axelsson P, Bratthall D (1984). The effect of a professional tooth-cleaning program on interdentally localized *Streptococcus mutans*. Caries Res 18:385–390.

Kristoffersson K, Axelsson P, Birkhed D, Bratthall D (1986). Caries prevalence, salivary *Streptococcus mutans* and dietary habits in 13-year-old Swedish schoolchildren. Commuity Dent Oral Epidemiol 1:9–16.

Kuusela S, Honkala E, Kannas L, Tynjala J, Wold B (1997). Oral hygiene habits of 11-year-olds in 22 European countries and Canada in 1993-94. J Dent Res 76:1602–1609.

Lang NP, Nyman S, Adler R, Joss A (1990). Absence of bleeding on probing. A predictor for periodontal health. J Clin Periodontol 17:714–721.

Lang NP, Karring T, eds (1994). Proceedings of the 1st European Workshop on Periodontology. Chicago: Quintessence.

Lindhe J, Hamp SE, Löe H (1973). Experimental periodontitis in the Beagle dog. J Periodontal Res 8: 1–10.

Lindskog BL, Zetterberg BL (1975). Swedish Medical Terminology. Almquist and Wiksell.

Lindskog S, Blomlöf L, Håkanson H (1994). Differential periodontal temperature measurements in the assessment of periodontal disease activity. An experimental and clinical activity. Scand J Dent Res 102:10–16.

Listgarten MA (1976). Structure of the microbial flora associated with periodontal health and disease in man. A light and electron microscopic study. J Periodontol 47:1–18.

Löe H, Theilade E, Jensen SB (1965). Experimental gingivitis in man. J Periodontol 36:177–187.

Löe H, von der Fehr FR, Schiött CR (1972). Inhibition of experimental caries by plaque prevention. The effect of chlorhexidine mouthrinses. Scand J Dent 80:1–9.

Löe H, Rindom Schiött C, Glavind L, Karring T (1976). 2 years' oral use of chlorhexidine in man. I. General design and clinical effects. J Periodontal Res 11:135–144.

Löe H, Ånerud Å, Boysen H, Smith M (1978). The natural history of periodontal disease in man. The rate of periodontal destruction before 40 years of age. J Periodontol 49:607–620.

Löe H, Kornman K (1982). Strategies in the use of antibacterial agents in periodontal disease. In: Genco RJ, Mergenhagen S (eds). Host–parasite Interactions in Periodontal Diseases. 376–381. Washington, DC: American Society for Microbiology.

Lövdal A, Arno A, Schei O, Waerhaug J (1961). Combined effect of subgingival scaling and controlled oral hygiene on the incidence of gingivitis. Acta Odontol Scand 19:537–555.

Lussi A (1991). Validity of diagnostic and treatment decisions of fissure caries. Caries Res 25:296–303.

Machtei EE, Dunford R, Hausmann E, Grossi SG, Powell J, Cummins D, Zambon JJ, Genco RJ (1997). Longitudinal study of prognostic factors in established periodontitis patients. J Clin Periodontol 24: 102–109.

Månsson B (1977). Caries progression in the first permanent molars. A longitudinal study. Swed Dent J 1:185–191.

Marsh PD (1989). Host defenses and microbila homeostasis: Role of microbial interactions. J Dent Res 68:1567–1575.

Marsh PD (1994). Microbial ecology of dental plaque and its significance in health and disease. Adv Dent Res 8(2):263–271.

Mejáre I, Malmgren B (1986). Clinical and radiographic appearance of proximal carious lesions at the time of operative treatment in young permanent teeth. Scand J Dent Res 94: 19–26.

Mejáre I, Mjör IA (1990). Glass ionomer and resin-based fissure sealants: A clinical study. Scand J Dent Res 98:345–350.

Michalowicz BS (1994a). People at risk for periodontitis—Genetic and heritable risk factors. J Periodontal Res 65:479–488.

Michalowicz BS (1994b). Genetic risk factors for periodontal diseases. Compend Contin Educ Dent 25:1036–1050.

Michalowicz BS, Aeppli D, Virag JG, Klump DG, Hinrichs JE, Segal NS, et al (1991a). Periodontal findings in adult twins. J Periodontol 62:293–299.

Michalowicz BS, Aeppli D, Kuba RK, Bereuter JE, Conry JP, Segal NL, et al (1991b). A twin study of gentic variation in proportional radiographic alveolar bone height. J Dent Res 70:1431–1435.

Miller WD (1984). The micro-organisms of the human mouth. The local and general diseases which are caused by them. 1890. Reprinted by S Karger, Basel, 1973.

Miyazaki H, Pilot T, Leclerq MH, Barnes D (1991a). Profiles of periodontal conditions in adolescents measured by CPITN. Int Dent J 41:67–73.

Miyazaki H, Pilot T, Leclerq MH, et al (1991b). Profiles of periodontal conditions in adults, measured by CPITN. Int Dent J 41:74–80.

Miyazaki H, Pilot T, Leclerq M-H (1992). Periodontal profiles. An overview of CPITN data in the WHO Global Oral Data Bank for the age group 15-19 years, 35-44 years and 65-75 years. Geneva: WHO.

Möller JJ, Poulsen S (1973). A standardized system for diagnosing, recording, and analyzing dental caries data. Scand J Dent Res 81:1–11.

Morch, T, Waerhaug J (1956) Quantitative evaluation of the effect of toothbrushing and toothpicking. J Periodontol 27:183.

Murray JJ (1969). Caries experience in 15-year-old children from fluoride and non-fluoride communities. Br Dent J 127:128–131.

Murray JJ, Rugg-Gunn AJ, Jenkins GN (1991). Fluorides and caries prevention, ed 3. Oxford: Butterworth-Heinemann.

Murray JJ, Rugg-Gunn AJ, Jenkins GN (1992). Fluorides in caries prevention, ed 3. London: Wright.

References

Norderyd O, Hugoson A, Grusovin G (1999). Risk for severe periodontal disease in a Swedish adult population. A longitudinal study. J Clin Periodontol 26 (in press).

Nyvad B, Fejerskov O (1986). Active root surface caries converted into inactive caries as a response to oral hygiene. Scand J Dent Res 94:281–284.

Øgaard B, Rölla G, Helgeland K (1983). Alkali-soluble and alkali-insoluble fluoride retention in demineralized enamel in vivo. Scand J Dent Res 91:200–204.

Øgaard B, Rölla G, Dijkman T, Ruben J, Arends J (1991). Effect of fluoride mouthrinsing on caries lesions development in shark enamel: An in situ model study. Scand J Dent Res 99:372–377.

Øgaard B, Cruz R, Rölla G (1992). Fluoride dentifrices, a possible cariostatic mechanism. In: Embery G, Rölla G (eds). Clinical and Biological Aspects of Dentifrices. New York: Oxford University Press.

O'Leary TJ, Drake RB, Naylor JE (1972). The plaque control record. J Periodontol 43:38–39.

Orland FJ, Blayney JR, Wendell-Harrison R (1954). Use of the germ-free animal technique in the study of experimental dental caries. J Dent Res 33:147–174.

Österberg T, Landt H (1976). Index for occlusal status. Tandlakärtidn 68:1216–1223.

Paulander J, Axelsson P, Lindhe J (1999). Relationship between level of education and oral health status in 35-, 50-, 65- and 75-year-olds. J Clin Periodontol (in press).

Petersson LG (1993). Fluoride mouthrinses and fluoride varnishes. Caries Res 27:35–42.

Petit MDA, van Steenbergen T, de Graaff J, van der Velden U (1993a). Transmission of Actinobacillus actinomycetemcomitans in families of adult periodontitis patients. J Periodontal Res 28:335–345.

Petit MDA, van Steenbergen T, de Graff J, van der Velden U (1993b). Epidemiology and transmission of *Porphyromonas gingivalis* and *Actinobacillus actinomycetemcomitans* among children and their family members. J Clin Periodontol 20:641–650.

Petit MDA, van Steenbergen TJM, Timmerman MF, de Graaff J, van der Velden U (1994). Prevalence of periodontitis and suspected periodontal pathogens in families of adult periodontitis patients. J Clin Periodontol 21:76–85.

Pitts NB, Rimmer PA (1992). An in vivo comparison of radiographic and directly assessed clinical caries status of posterior approximal surfaces in primary and permanent teeth. Caries Res 26:146–152.

Preus HR, Zambon JJ, Dunford RG, Genco RJ (1994). The distribution and transmission of *Actinobacillus actinomycetemcomitans* in families with established adult periodontitis. J Periodontol 65:2–7.

Ramberg P, Lindhe J, Dahlén G, Volpe AR (1994). The influence of gingival inflammation on de novo plaque formation. J Clin Periodontol 21:51–56.

Ramberg P, Axelsson P, Lindhe J (1995a). Plaque formation at healthy and inflamed gingival sites in young individuals. J Clin Periodontol 22 (1):85–88.

Ramberg P, Furuichi Y, Sherl D, Volpe AR, Nabi N, Gaffar A, Lindhe J (1995b). The effect of triclosan on developing gingivitis. J Clin Periodontol 22(6): 442–448.

Ravald N, Birkhed D (1991). Factors associated with active and inactive root caries in patients with periodontal disease. Caries Res 25:377–384.

Ravald N (1992). Studies on root surface caries in patients with periodontal disease [thesis]. Göteborg: University of Göteborg.

Richards A, Banting DW (1996). Fluoride toothpastes. In: Fejerskov O, Ekstrand J, Burt B. Fluoride in Dentistry. Copenhagen: Munksgaard.

Ripa LW (1993). Sealants revisited: An update of the effectiveness of pit and fissure sealants. Caries Res 27(Suppl 1):77–82.

Ritz L, Hefti AF, Rateitschak KH (1992). An in vitro investigation on the loss of substance in scaling with various instruments. J Clin Periodontol 18:643–647.

Rosling B (1976). Plaque control. A determining factor in the treatment of periodontal disease [thesis]. Gothenburg: University of Gothenburg.

Saarela M, Stucki A-M, von Troil-Lindén B, Alaluusua S, Jousimies-Somer H, Asikainen S (1993c). Intra- and interindividual comparison of *Porphyromonas gingivalis* genotypes. FEMS Immunol Med Microbiol 6:99–102.

Saxer UP, Mühlemann HR (1975). Motivation und Aufklärung. Schweiz Monatsschr Zahnheilk 85: 905–919.

Scheie A (1994). Mechanisms of dental plaque formation. Adv Dent Res 8:246–253.

Schroers K (1994). A controlled clinical study on the effect of Bifluorid 12 on sensitive root surfaces [in German]. Abstract.

Seppä L (1994). Fluoride release and effect on enamel softening by fluoride-treated and fluoride-untreated glass-ionomer specimens. Caries Res 28: 406–408.

Silness J, Löe H (1964). Periodontal disease in pregnancy. II. Correlation between oral hygiene and periodontal condition. Acta Odontol Scand 22: 121–135.

Sjödin B, Crossner C, Unell L, Östlund P (1989). A retrospective radiographic study of alveolar bone loss in the primary dentition in patients with localized juvenile periodontitis. J Clin Periodontol 16: 124–127.

Sjödin B, Matsson L, Unell L, Egelberg J (1993). Marginal bone loss in the primary dentition of patients with juvenile periodontitis. J Clin Periodontol 20:32–36.

Socransky SS, Haffajee AD, Goodson JM, Lindhe J (1984). New concepts of destructive periodontal disease. J Clin Periodontol 11(1):21–32.

Stephen KW, Boyle IT, Campbell D, McNee S, Boyle P (1984). Five-year fluoridated milk study in Scotland. Comm Dent Oral Epidemiol 12:223–229.

Ten Cate JM, Van Duinen R (1995). Hypermineralization of dental lesions adjacent to glass-ionomer cement restorations. J Dent Res 74:1266–1271.

Ten Cate JM, Featherstone J (1996). Physicochemical aspects of fluoride-enamel interactions. In: Fejerskov O, Ekstrand J, Burt B (eds). Fluoride in Dentistry. Copenhagen: Munksgaard.

Theilade E, Wright W, Jensen B, Loe H (1966). Experimental gingivitis in man. II. A longitudinal clinical and bacteriological investigation. J Periodontal Res 1:1–13.

Theilade E, Theilade J (1976). Role of plaque in the etiology of periodontal disease and caries. Oral Sci Rev 9:23.

Thylstrup A, Fejerskov O (1978). Clinical appearance of dental fluorosis in permanent teeth in relation to histological changes. Community Dent Oral Epidemiol 6:315–328.

Thylstrup A, Fejerskov O (1994). Clinical and pathological features of dental caries. 111–157. In: Thylstrup A, Fejerskov O (eds). Textbook of Clinical Cariology. Copenhagen: Munksgaard.

Thylstrup A, Vinther D, Christiansen J (1997). Promoting changes in clinical practice. Treatment time and outcome studies in a Danish public child dental health clinic. Community Dent Oral Epidemiol 25:126–134.

Tonetti MS, Pino-Prato G, Cortellini P (1995). Effect of cigarette smoking on periodontal healing following GTR in infrabony defects. A preliminary retrospective study. J Clin Periodontol 22:229–234.

Torell P, Ericsson Y (1965). Two-year test with different methods of local caries-preventive fluoride application in Swedish schoolchildren. Acta Odontol Scand 23:287–322.

Van der Weijden GA, Timmerman M, Danser M, Van der Velden U (1998). The role of automated toothbrushes. In: Lang NP (ed). Proceedings of the European Workshop on Mechanical Plaque Control. Chicago: Quintessence, 138–155.

Van Dyke TE, Lavine MJ, Genco RJ (1987). Neutrophil function and oral disease. J Oral Pathol 14:95–120.

Van Steenbergen TJM, Petit MD, Scholte LE, van der Velden U, de Graaf J (1993). Transmission of Porphyromonas gingivalis between spouses. J Clin Periodontol 20:340–345.

Van Winkelhoff AJ, Rams TE, Slots J (1996). Systemic antibiotic therapy in periodontics. Periodontol 2000 10:45–78.

Volpe AR, Petrone ME, Davies RM (1993). A critical review of the 10 pivotal caries clinical studies used in a recent meta-analysis comparing the anticaries efficacy of sodium fluoride and sodium monofluorophosphate dentifrice. Am J Dent 6:13–42.

Von der Fehr FT, Löe H, Theilade E (1970). Experimental caries in man. Caries Res 4:131–148.

Von Troil-Lindén B, Torkko H, Alaluusua S, Wolf J, Jousimies-Somer H, Asikainen S (1995). Periodontal findings in spouses. A clinical, radiographic and microbiological study. J Clin Periodontol 22:93–99.

Waerhaug J (1981a). Effect of toothbrushing on subgingival plaque formation. J Periodontol 52:30–34.

Waerhaug J (1981b). Healing of the dento-epithelial junction following the use of dental floss. J Clin Periodontol 8:144–150.

Weatherell JA, Deutsch D, Robinson C, Hallsworth AS (1977). Assimilation of fluoride by enamel throughout the life of the tooth. Caries Res 11:85–115.

Weinstein P, Getz I (1978). Changing human behavior—strategies for preventive dentistry. Science Research Association (SRA) Inc.

Wendt LK, Koch G (1988). Fissure sealant in permanent first molars after 10 years. Swed Dent J 12:181–185.

Wendt LK, Hallonsten A, Koch G, Birkhed D (1994). Oral hygiene in relation to caries development and immigrant status in infants and toddlers. Scand J Dent Res 102:269–273.

Zambon JJ, Christersson LA, Slots J (1983). *Actinobacillus actinomycetemcomitans* in human periodontal disease. Prevalence in patient groups and distribution of biotypes and serotypes within families. J Periodontol 54:707–711.

Zambon JJ, Grossi S, Machtei E, et al (1996). Cigarette smoking increases the risk for subgingival infection with periodontal pathogens. J Periodontol (Suppl) 67:1050–1054.

Zickert I, Lindvall AM, Axelsson P (1982). Effect on caries and gingivitis of a preventive program based on oral hygiene measures and fluoride application. Community Dent Oral Epidemiol 10:289–295.

LIST OF ABBREVIATIONS USED

APITN—Apical Periodontal Index of Treatment Needs
AN(U)G—acute necrotizing ulcerative gingivitis
ARPP—adult rapidly progressive periodontitis
ACP—adult (chronic) periodontitis
AP—adult periodontitis
ART—atraumatic restorative technique

CCITN—Community Caries Index of Treatment Needs
CEJ—cementoenamel junction
CHX—chlorhexidine
CN(U)G—chronic necrotizing ulcerative gingivitis
CPITN—Community Periodontal Index of Treatment Needs

EOP—early onset periodontitis

FA—fluorapatite
FDI—Fédération Dentaire Internationale

GBI—Gingival Bleeding Index
GC—glass-ionomer cement
GJP—generalized juvenile periodontitis
GODB—Global Oral Data Bank
GPJP—generalized postjuvenile periodontitis
GPP—generalized prepubertal periodontitis

HA—hydroxyapatite

LBC—lactobacillus count
LJP—localized juvenile periodontitis
LPJP—localized postjuvenile periodontitis
LPP—localized prepubertal periodontitis

MS—mutans streptococci

NP—necrotizing periodontitis

OR—odds ratio

PBI—papilla bleeding index
PCPC—professional chemical plaque control
PFRI—Plaque Formation Rate Index
PI—Plaque Index
PMNL—polymorphonuclear leukocytes
PMTC—professional mechanical toothcleaning
PRF—prognostic risk factors

RF—risk factors
RI—risk indicators

SFR—salivary flow rate

WHO—World Health Organization
  EURO—Regional Office Europe
  EMRO—Regional Office Eastern Mediterranean
  AMRO—Regional Office America
  AFRO—Regional Office Africa
  WPRO—Regional Office Western Pacific
  SEARO—Regional Office Southeastern Asia